Sweet Mary Jane

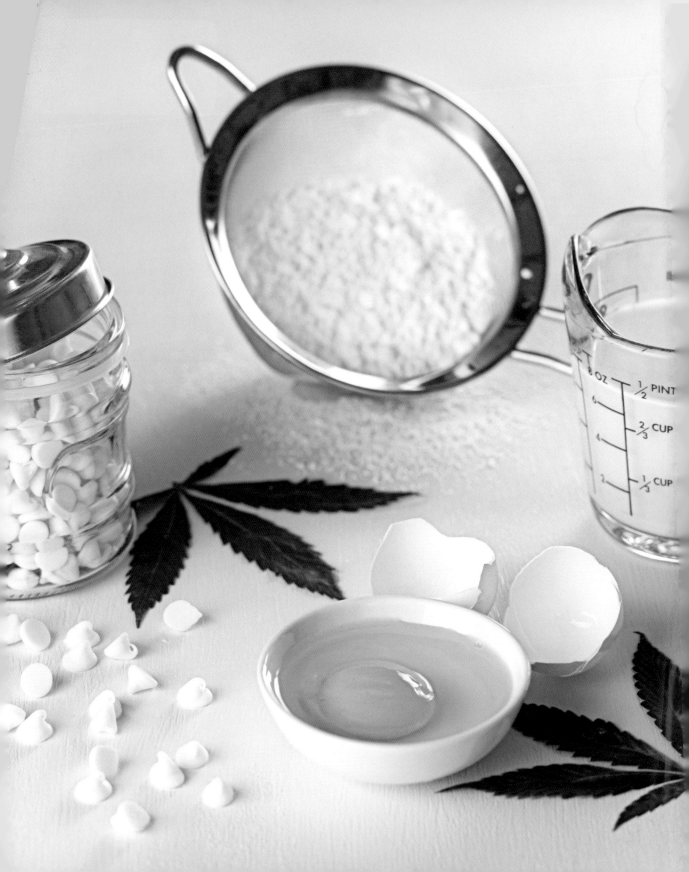

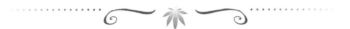

Sweet Mary Jane

75 DELICIOUS CANNABIS-INFUSED

HIGH-END DESSERTS

KARIN LAZARUS

AVERY

AN IMPRINT OF PENGUIN RANDOM HOUSE

NEW YORK

AVERY

An imprint of Penguin Random House, LLC
375 Hudson Street
New York, New York 10014

Appendix A chart courtesy of Gaetano Iannoccone.

Most Avery books are available at special quantity discounts for bulk purchase for sales promotions,
premiums, fund-raising, and educational needs. For details, write
Special.Markets@penguinrandomhouse.com.

Library of Congress Cataloging-in-Publication Data

Lazarus, Karin.
Sweet Mary Jane : 75 delicious cannabis-infused high-end desserts / Karin Lazarus.
p.   cm.
ISBN 978-1-58333-565-9
1. Cooking (Marijuana)   2. Desserts.   I. Title.
TX819.M25L39   2015   2014047004
641.86—dc23

Printed in the United States of America
1   3   5   7   9   10   8   6   4   2

BOOK DESIGN BY AMANDA DEWEY

For my mom, who taught me to believe in myself

Contents

INTRODUCTION *1*

Health Benefits from Cannabis *15*

Equipment, Measurements, and Terms *21*

Ingredients *29*

Infusions *35*

Brownies and Bars *57*

Cookies *87*

Cakes and Sweet Breads *121*

Cupcakes and Muffins *143*

Tarts and Pastries *169*

Ice Creams and Sorbets *191*

Puddings and Flans *207*

Creative Bites *217*

Truffles *255*

Sauces *271*

APPENDIX A: MEDICINAL USES FOR CANNABINOIDS *279*

APPENDIX B: ONLINE RESOURCES *281*

ACKNOWLEDGMENTS *283*

INDEX *285*

Sweet Mary Jane

Introduction

Our kitchen in Boulder, Colorado, sits quietly among the foothills of the Front Range, far from a main road. We don't have a big sign that shows people where to find us; as a matter of fact, we don't have any sign at all. You need to enter a security code to get inside in the morning, and set it again when you leave at night. Some people might find this unusual, having to bake under security cameras that watch you 24/7, and, truthfully, at first it *was* a bit strange for all of us in the kitchen. But now we don't even think about it.

I'm Karin Lazarus, founder of Sweet Mary Jane Bakery. I've been baking since I was eight, when my mom gave me a Sunbeam Mixmaster and a Betty Crocker cookbook. My mother kept our family's pantry stocked with all the goodies Hostess had to offer, plus what she herself baked. We ate sweet treats all the time: homemade chocolate pudding with toasted walnuts and a dollop of freshly whipped cream, Linzer cookies filled with raspberry preserves and dusted with powdered sugar, icebox cookie cake, and chocolate chip cookies baked at the drop of a hat, just because. She'd even top homemade waffles with a big scoop of vanilla ice cream and pure maple syrup. That got me out of bed in the morning! I had the biggest sweet tooth in the universe, and my mom made sure I could satisfy it. But even back then, I wanted to make things on my own.

After baking my very first batch of chocolate chip cookies, my family's *oob*s and *abb*s were such a thrill. Oh, I was hooked. I was a Girl Scout, and of course I sold Girl Scout cookies, but as I was delivering boxes to the neighbors, I fantasized about having made the cookies myself. In the summertime, while other kids set up lemonade stands, I opened a *cookie* stand. Baking, I saw, was not only fun but profitable. Best of all, it made people happy.

That's what I've aimed to do ever since.

In high school, I baked for head shops in New York City—you know, those funky little stores that sell hippie clothing, incense and perfume (patchouli!), and drug paraphernalia. Way back then, it was uninfused goodies, things like rose petal sweet bread, banana bread, peach bread, and assorted cookies and brownies. I doubt I made enough money to cover the ingredients, but I didn't care; I loved doing it. I baked all through college, too, for family gatherings and also for friends. Nobody I knew ever went without a birthday cake. I made delicious treats for when the munchies struck, and took special requests for party desserts. I was thrilled that people wanted me to bake for them.

I married after graduation, and moved to New York with my husband, Charley. My degree was in photography and I immediately found work as an artists' representative. Although I enjoyed the job (and it certainly paid the bills), it wasn't something I felt passionate about. I wanted a business of my own, and I knew it had to revolve around cooking. So I signed up for catering classes in Chelsea. This covered both cooking and the business end of things, and it was great fun. Living in the city, I was surrounded by wonderful restaurants and—especially important, given my sweet tooth!—bakeries: Dean & DeLuca, Vesuvio Italian Bakery, The Silver Palate, Chelsea Market. There was a tiny Italian place across from our apartment on Sullivan Street, and I used to walk over and get the best biscotti before heading to work. During Lent, they made hot cross buns and sold them toasty warm and slathered with fresh, creamy butter, and there were lines of happy customers out the door. Owning a bakery, I thought, must be the best thing in the world.

A few years later, my husband and I moved to Tortola in the British Virgin Islands. White sand, hot sun, the beautiful sea. Charley worked as a builder while I kept busy with private catering jobs, parties for locals and for the tourists who come to the Caribbean to sail. Once our daughter, Lucienne, was born, however, we decided that it was time to return to reality—we wanted to raise her in the States. We lived again for a while in New York, then moved to Boulder, Colorado, and after some years, I found myself a single mom. This coincided with a faltering economy. Work was hard to come by. I wrote and tested recipes for a healthy lifestyle magazine, which I loved doing, although the pay was modest and it was difficult to make ends meet. Then I met a wonderful food stylist who taught me the tricks of that trade, but here in Boulder there is not much call for that sort of work. Also, I wanted to be baking and having people eat the food, not just making it look beautiful while rendering it inedible with styling tricks. So while these jobs kept me afloat and provided valuable experience, I was still dreaming my bakery dream.

Making confections is an art form. Every aspect of the process requires creative attention, from deciding what to bake to the final product. I love sifting flour, creaming together butter and sugar, adding in fragrant extracts and a pinch of salt. I love the comforting scents that fill the kitchen, and the thrill of coming up with clever garnishes. I especially love that magical moment when you pull a baking sheet from the oven and know that what you've made is absolutely perfect.

I am forever dreaming up new creations. Inspiration is everywhere. It might be a new ingredient I've just seen in a store or online (Himalayan pink salt!), or a particular combination of flavors that I've never tried, like caramel corn, blueberries, ice cream, and peanut butter. Retro desserts inspired confections like our Carrot Cake Cookies (page 93), while more modern tastes led me down the road to Chai High Truffles (page 259). The change of seasons is always a fine time for discovering and celebrating new tastes. I look for comfort in winter, brightness for spring. Summer is for cool and refreshing sensations. Warming flavors make fall feel festive.

Our day in the kitchen begins early. We check orders, preheat the ovens, melt chocolates, and bring butter and eggs to room temperature. Everything is measured, ready to go before the baking process begins; this is known as *mise en place*. Proper *mise en place* ensures that all your equipment and ingredients are on hand the second they are needed in a recipe, and also ensures that you won't forget to add an ingredient. The brownies are in the oven, baking away, the sweet scent of chocolate filling the air, and then you get a sinking feeling that you may have forgotten to add the sugar. . . . We've all been there.

Once preparations have been properly made, we bake. We make frostings and dip confections. We package and label. Signature desserts, such as our award-winning OMG! Brownie Cheesecake Bars (page 73) and Key Lime Kickers (page 261), are always on the order board.

At the end of the day, we lock up just like any other business. But at night, an armed security guard watches out for the treasures inside our door. Because we are not just any old bakery: Sweet Mary Jane is a medical marijuana bakery.

The idea of opening a marijuana bakery snuck up on me so quietly I can't say exactly when and how it took hold. In the mid-2000s, *Weeds*, a series about a widowed suburban mom who sold marijuana to survive, became a sensation on cable TV. I read an article about the health benefits of cannabis, watched a few news reports on medical marijuana dispensaries in California. Although I hadn't used marijuana in years, I became intrigued with the idea that this plant could improve lives. I'd known since high school, of course, that cannabis could be baked into treats—remember the pot brownies in *I Love You, Alice B. Toklas*? But now, for the first time, I thought about starting a business that combined medical marijuana with my love of baking.

I knew that Colorado's Amendment 20, passed in 2002, allowed for legal possession of marijuana for medical purposes, but the amounts permitted were small—no more than two ounces—and the amendment applied only to qualifying patients or caregivers. In 2007, a Colorado judge had overturned the required five-patients-to-one-caregiver ratio, opening the door to wider sales, but there was always a fear of prosecution, especially at the federal level. A theoretical problem, in my case, as I had no startup money.

Toward the end of 2009, with my daughter off at college, I traveled to Tortola for an extended visit. I was, at that time, in the habit of sending recipes in to cooking contests, and before I left, I entered my Chocolate-Filled Pandan Dumplings in TuttiFoodie—Scharffen Berger's Chocolate Adventure Contest. Then I promptly forgot about it—winning a recipe contest is like winning the lottery: largely a fantasy. The following spring I learned that I'd won the $10,000 grand prize. I jumped for joy. (Seriously, I *jumped*, laughing and screaming, "*I did it!*" You can watch a video of the judge, Chef Elizabeth Falkner, making the recipe on my website, www.ilovesmj.com. It's delicious, by the way.) Suddenly, I had startup money.

Meanwhile, the laws in Colorado had changed. With the passage of HB-1284 in 2010, commercial dispensaries, grow operations, and the manufacture of edibles became fully legal. What I'd always thought was a good idea now seemed like a great one.

From Tortola, I excitedly called dispensaries and spoke with owners. There have always been people selling, baking, and growing marijuana, but they mostly operated underground; you wouldn't find them on a member list at the local Chamber of Commerce. I had so many questions for these intrepid souls. What kind of people used medical marijuana? What specific conditions did it help? And what was the best way to administer the drug? Everyone was friendly and supportive and said that I should come see them when I returned to the States. I got on a plane, thinking happily, *Now I can start my bakery.*

Back in Colorado, I read everything I could get my hands on about cannabis. I'd always been interested in fresh and healthy eating, but now this interest took on urgency. I learned about the specific healing properties of cannabinoids, how they match *endo*cannabinoids, compounds produced naturally by our own bodies. Cannabinoids affect a range of human physiological processes; among other things, they help balance mood, alter the perception of pain, and can positively affect appetite and memory. (See Health Benefits from Cannabis, page 15; see also Appendix A on page 279 for a handy chart, and Appendix B on page 281 for a list of websites that provide further information.)

I applied for a Red Card. (Red Cards are issued by the Colorado Department of Health and Environment to residents over the age of eighteen, and are required to purchase medical marijuana.) Then I visited dispensaries. I hoped to learn as much as I could about the business, which was then in its infancy. I spoke with owners and met many patients. It was eye-opening, hearing how cannabis had changed their daily lives. In addition to smokable weed, most dispensaries stocked edibles: store-bought wafer cookies made into sandwich cookies with a homemade, infused-cream filling; chocolate brownies; lollipops and gummies. I knew there was a market. But without a solid industry history to examine, there were no proven formulas for how to run such an operation, no guidelines for how to bake properly with marijuana, or to grow.

I worked on a business plan for the bakery. This was loosely drawn at first and for my eyes only, but eventually I showed it around. My parents were supportive from the get-go. They lived in New York City, and at first couldn't fathom that marijuana was legal in Colorado—they were worried that I might somehow be arrested; every time we spoke on the phone, they told me how proud they were of me for being brave. (My dad passed away in 2012, and I so wish he could have seen this book, and that I'm still not in jail!) My daughter, Lucienne, who was in her sophomore year at George Washington University, became my greatest support. Each time she returned to Colorado, she helped with ideas for the menu and names for products. (Once she graduated, she came back to Boulder for good, and she is now part of the family business.)

Early on, a handful of friends stood behind me. Others thought I was crazy. "You're going to put all that prize money into . . . weed?!" The idea *was* challenging. And the more I investigated the nitty-gritty of the business, the more daunting it seemed. For one thing, opening a marijuana bakery meant dealing with government bureaucracies.

Obtaining a Marijuana Infused Products license is the first step to opening a bakery. The application requires proof of residence, and you must give verifiable addresses for the previous five years. You must provide a detailed financial history, including bank and credit card statements and tax returns, and state where the money to fund the business will come from. You must also disclose your arrest record, if you have one, and the details of any bankruptcy proceedings, and you must be fingerprinted. And *before* you do any of this, you must have already secured a location for your business, either buying or renting, and it must be legal to run a marijuana business out of this space. Then you must prove legal possession of the premises to the state, and give them a diagram of your space showing where everything—refrigerators, ovens, cabinets, and countertops—will go, including the cameras. Then there are the fees! And oh, by the way, be prepared, because the rules change all the time. Rules about labeling, state-mandated warnings and recommended doses, THC (the active ingredient in marijuana) levels, how many doses are in each product, how exactly it has been infused, and which plant the marijuana came from.

It was overwhelming—I was overwhelmed.

So I set aside the business plan for a while. I asked myself a question: *Why* did I want to open a marijuana bakery? To answer it, I followed my heart. I went back into the kitchen and baked.

Here I'd like to give a shout-out to those anonymous, adventurous souls who first realized we could bake brownies with weed. What a spectacular idea. Back in the good old days (or maybe they were the bad old days?), you'd choke down an over-baked brownie flecked with bits of something that tasted like lawn clippings. But I knew it was possible to create confections that would be like portals to our fondest memories. I didn't want to make "stoner food." I wanted to bake as I would for a regular bakery, making beautiful treats that tasted as good as they looked.

I started small, testing infusing processes and recipes in my own home kitchen and giving away the results to friends.

The first treat I made was a brownie called Walnut Fantasy (page 83). I'd been baking this brownie forever without weed, and knew it was delicious, so it was relatively simple to tweak the recipe and turn it into an infused treat. My taste-testers loved it. Next up was a brownie called Merciful (page 69), with four kinds of chocolate—semisweet, unsweetened, cocoa powder, and white chocolate. This was also a hit. From there, I moved off the brownie path, adding True Confections (a bite-size peanut-butter-and-pretzel confection wrapped in a cloak of semisweet chocolate—check out page 251) and Pop Star Caramel Corn (which is exactly as it sounds—see page 246). I was very lucky; not only were these early treats a success, but they remain some of our most popular items.

Some things didn't work. I failed at making plain chocolates—I never could get the texture right (I'm going to keep trying!). Meringue cookies failed multiple times (though eventually I figured it out), and it took me forever to learn how to make truffles. At first I infused them with hash, but the flavor was all wrong.

I learned as I baked. The taste and color of cannabis can be overpowering. Who wants to eat a green cookie? (To be honest, some people like the flavor. I'm just not one of them.) Fruit, chocolate, coffee, peanut butter, and vanilla are all ingredients that mask the flavor of weed, but with infused butter or coconut oil, you will still taste the cannabis. That's when I got the idea of infusing granulated white sugar. It changed everything. Infused sugar is magical, with barely a hint of weed in the finished product. This opened the door to further experiments, ways to bring in flavors and textures associated with the holidays, with the finale of a celebratory meal, with sneaking into the kitchen in the middle of the night for a delectable reward.

After testing so many recipes, my faith in the bakery dream was restored. It was finally time to look for kitchen space, which turned out to be no easy task. Imagine calling a landlord and asking if you can set up shop in his space selling weed. Landlords and real estate agents hung up on me when I told them what I was looking for. Then I met a fabulous real estate agent who not only used weed herself but was enthusiastic about the business. She found me the space I am in today. (Thank you, Cathy!)

I applied for and received licenses from both the state of Colorado and Boulder County, built out a small commercial kitchen, and installed a used home oven purchased at a thrift store for sixty dollars—it was only a few steps above my old Easy Bake Oven! In went stainless-steel tables and sinks, a freezer, and refrigerators from a restaurant supply company that sold used equipment.

All the while, I continued to create recipes. I baked and baked and baked. There is a meditative quality to baking in general, but with this kind of product I thought a lot about who might buy it and the medical conditions they would be hoping to treat. I thought about what flavors and ingredients would work well with weed. I made sure that the dosing was always correct. My goal from the beginning has been to produce baked goods that are healthful and beautiful, both to eat and to behold.

Once I had a good selection of products, I packaged up sample goodie bags and brought them to as many dispensaries as I could. I hoped the owners would try them, but nine times out of ten, the goodies disappeared before that could happen. (I wonder where they went?) So I'd start all over again, persisting, until eventually the goods reached the right people. All our baked items are infused with a hefty dose of THC, and soon orders trickled in. I had just enough money to keep myself going, not one penny more, but patients told other patients, and dispensary owners spread the word. Sweet Mary Jane began to take off.

Today, Sweet Mary Jane is a household name in Colorado's medical marijuana community. We have twelve employees, a dream team without which the bakery would not exist. This includes bakers, concentrate makers, and a delivery crew. We don't advertise—we never have—yet the kitchen is always hopping. We sell to more than one hundred dispensaries all over Colorado, sending out more than two thousand delightfully infused treats every week.

What sets us apart is a commitment to making the highest-quality products possible. It starts with ingredients—premium cannabis, good chocolates, real butter, pure vanilla—and continues with our process: Our methods of baking have been carefully thought out, honed, and refined. Orders are custom made. Brownies, for example, are made in small batches. It's the only way to achieve that rich, melt-in-your-mouth texture.

This attention to detail has paid off. In April 2013, Sweet Mary Jane won the first-place trophy in the Rooster THC Classic for our OMG! Brownie Cheesecake Bars. In November 2013, we took home two first-place awards in the Hemp Connoisseur THC Championship for our Key Lime Kickers. Both recipes are in this cookbook.

One top priority at the bakery now is keeping up with regulations. All employees at Sweet Mary Jane wear government-issued ID badges, received after completing an application that includes fingerprinting and a full background check by the Marijuana Enforcement Division. In 2014, marijuana businesses in Colorado went on to the Marijuana Inventory Tracking System, which tracks products from seed to sale. Every plant and every unit of processed product—whether buds or marijuana-infused treats—must have a radio frequency identification tag attached to it; these are tracked by satellite. Every package sent to a dispensary is batch-numbered and packaged with strict warning labels, and we report every single infused item that leaves or comes into the kitchen. This helps the state ensure that items come from authorized sources.

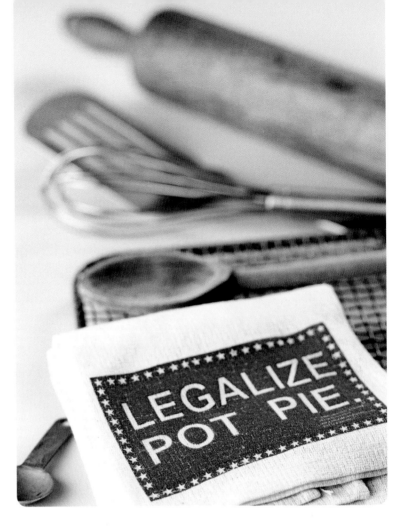

Our biggest problem these days is cash. Not the lack of it, which handicaps so many small businesses, but what to do with the actual physical *cash*. It is still a bit like the old Wild West here. Because the sale of weed remains illegal at the federal level, we in the industry cannot bank our money. Many of us have employees to pay, and vendors, and of course we must pay our taxes. And obviously, handling large amounts of cash is dangerous. Safe-deposit boxes, armed guards, and security cameras are all a part of daily life.

In 2014, Colorado decided to address this problem, and there has been encouraging talk of creating a cannabis co-op. Colorado lawmakers have already approved the world's first banking system designed to accommodate the marijuana industry. Governor John Hickenlooper has signed the bill. But the Federal Reserve must give its blessing before the bill's provisions can take effect. We shall see.

The rules for staying compliant change all the time, but that's okay. Legal marijuana is new. We're all learning. The only thing I know for sure is to expect the unexpected.

I wouldn't trade what I'm doing for anything. For all the challenges of this business, the rewards are greater. Every time a patient calls Sweet Mary Jane to tell me how much their symptoms have been helped by one of our products, I feel an uncontainable joy.

The confection business is sweet.

A Note from Karin

There are tricks to baking with cannabis, referred to throughout this cookbook as *bud*, *weed*, or *marijuana*. All that stands between you and a fabulous, infused, homestyle-with-a-twist confection is know-how. In the pages that follow, I will teach you the secrets of creating sophisticated desserts and cult favorites. You will use natural, whole foods and fresh, adventurous ingredients to create goodies that are good for you and a pleasure to eat.

Before you start, please read the Infusions chapter (all the way through!) on pages 35 to 55 to make sure you understand dosing. Do not bake one single thing until you do. I mean it.

I recommend that you also read through Health Benefits from Cannabis (page 15); Equipment, Measurements, and Terms (page 21); and Ingredients (page 29). There's no such thing as being "too well informed."

Begin with the recipes for the lowest dosages of Buddha Budda, Coconut Bliss, or

Hey Sugar! (pages 43, 46, and 51, respectively). Always wait two hours before taking another dose; edibles can take a while to kick in. (Please see page 17 for the major differences between oral and edible cannabis.) And remember: These confections look *exactly* like something you'd find in a bakery, while being emphatically *only* for the twenty-one-and-over crowd. So **KEEP OUT OF REACH OF CHILDREN**.

Cookbook authors will almost always tell you to taste as you are cooking, but I am telling you *not* to. We all love to taste the batter, but please don't do that with these recipes. (Put down that cookie dough!) Either bake the dessert uninfused, to see if you like the flavors, or bake an infused dessert and taste it *after* you have divided it into doses. Every single dessert in this book can be made uninfused; just substitute regular butter, coconut oil, or sugar for the infused versions. And a final word of warning here: If you cook with weed, your kitchen *will* smell like weed.

I think that's everything I wanted to tell you. And so . . .

Bakers, start your ovens!

Health Benefits
from Cannabis

The recent legalization of marijuana in Colorado and other states opens the door to increased investigation into the medicinal properties of cannabis, one of the most powerful healing plants on the planet. Important research has been conducted by Dr. Raphael Mechoulam ("the man who discovered THC"), an Israeli professor of medicinal chemistry at the Hebrew University of Jerusalem; by scientists at the Center for Medicinal Cannabis Research at the University of California, San Diego; and by Dr. William Courtney at Cannabis International. Dr. Sanjay Gupta, CNN's chief medical correspondent, has written of cannabis, "It doesn't have a high potential for abuse, and there are very legitimate medical applications. In fact, sometimes marijuana is the only thing that works."

Difficulties remain, however, as federal regulations still classify marijuana as a Schedule I substance.

Two federal agencies, the Drug Enforcement Administration and the Food and Drug Administration, call the shots on which substances are added or removed from the various schedules. The system has five categories. Factors that determine which category a drug falls into are whether a given drug has the potential for severe psychological and/or physical dependence, and also whether there is a high potential for abuse. Schedule I drugs are the most dangerous class. As the number goes up— Schedule II, Schedule III, etc.—the abuse potential goes down, with Schedule V drugs (things like cough preparations with less than 200 milliliters of codeine) having the least potential for abuse.

Under this system, heroin and cannabis, as Schedule I drugs, are equally dangerous (other Schedule I drugs are LSD, Ecstasy, and peyote), while methamphetamine, a Schedule II drug, is classified as being *less* dangerous than marijuana. It is hard to see how this makes sense. The classification of marijuana as a Schedule I drug makes it particularly difficult for cannabis researchers to design and fund their studies. But where there's a will, there's a way. In September 2014, I attended the Marijuana for Medical Professionals Conference in Denver. Panels were lively, and enthusiasm remains high. Many researchers are moving forward with private funding, and some are even financing studies out of their own pockets. Video-conferenced in for a talk titled "Cannabis Medicine in Perspective," Dr. Lester Grinspoon, professor emeritus at Harvard University, author of several books about the medical use of marijuana, and founding editor of the *Harvard Mental Health Letter*, said, "I can't wait to get to Colorado to breathe the air of freedom."

The movement to have marijuana reclassified is growing. Organizations that work on behalf of this cause include NORML (http://norml.org), Sensible Colorado (http://sensiblecolorado.org), and Marijuana Policy Project (http://www.mpp.org).

In the meantime, people from all over the United States have been moving to Colorado in order to use cannabis as part of their treatment protocol. I can't even begin to count the number of patients who have called Sweet Mary Jane to thank us for the relief our edibles has given them.

Cannabis is an antioxidant. It is anti-inflammatory and neuroprotective. Studies have shown that it can slow the spread of cancer; prevent or lessen opiate addiction; and combat depression, PTSD, anxiety, and ADHD. It can help with the management of Crohn's disease, as it plays a role in limiting intestinal inflammation. Cannabis is also useful in treating epilepsy and other seizure disorders, MS, muscle spasms, restless leg syndrome, and Tourette's syndrome. It can reduce blood pressure; treat glaucoma; alleviate pain, arthritis, and fibromyalgia; and inhibit HIV. It is also linked to lower insulin levels in diabetics. The cannabinoids found in the plant deliver important palliative effects, and some patients have been able to get off other medications and use only cannabis to treat their symptoms, with far fewer side effects.

Finally, there are studies that indicate that THC (the primary psychoactive substance) and CBD (the main non-psychoactive ingredient) display anti-convulsive properties in animals, and thus may limit neurological damage from concussions and strokes. According to Dr. Tim England, honorary consultant stroke physician at the University of Nottingham and Royal Derby Hospital, the chemical compounds found in cannabis may shrink the area of the brain affected by stroke. Cannabinoids may also help improve overall brain function following a stroke.

WHY ORAL CANNABIS IS DIFFERENT

Edibles can be a healthier alternative to inhaled cannabis. Some patients, such as those on supplemental oxygen, turn to edibles as a healthier option to inhaling smoke.

Inhaled cannabinoids are delivered to the bloodstream through the lungs. Once in the bloodstream, they become available to the brain and central nervous system. Inhalation is the fastest method of delivery, with peak blood levels achieved within twenty minutes and lasting for up to two hours, depending on the strain and grade of cannabis. Oral ingestion is slower, because the cannabinoids must go through the gastrointestinal tract before entering the bloodstream. Cannabinoids are released in waves as they are processed by the stomach, and slowly digested, providing up to eight hours of relief.

During the decarboxylation and cooking process, inactive cannabinoids, such as THC-A and CBD-A, are converted to THC and CBD, which work together, providing effective treatment for many disorders.

With edibles, there is reduced throat and lung irritation, and the longer duration results in a less frequent need to re-dose. For cancer patients suffering from nausea caused by their treatments, and for patients with eating and digestive disorders, edibles are not only a great source of nausea-reducing CBDs but a vital source of nutrients and calories.

My love of baking is what got me started in this industry, but what keeps me going is the patients. I'd read about the healing powers of cannabis, but didn't know how people would react to our confections. And yet, every day, Sweet Mary Jane receives calls from patients thanking us for all we have done to alleviate their symptoms.

See Appendix A on page 279 for a chart listing the various cannabinoids and their properties.

See Appendix B on page 281 for websites that contain further information about the health benefits of cannabinoids.

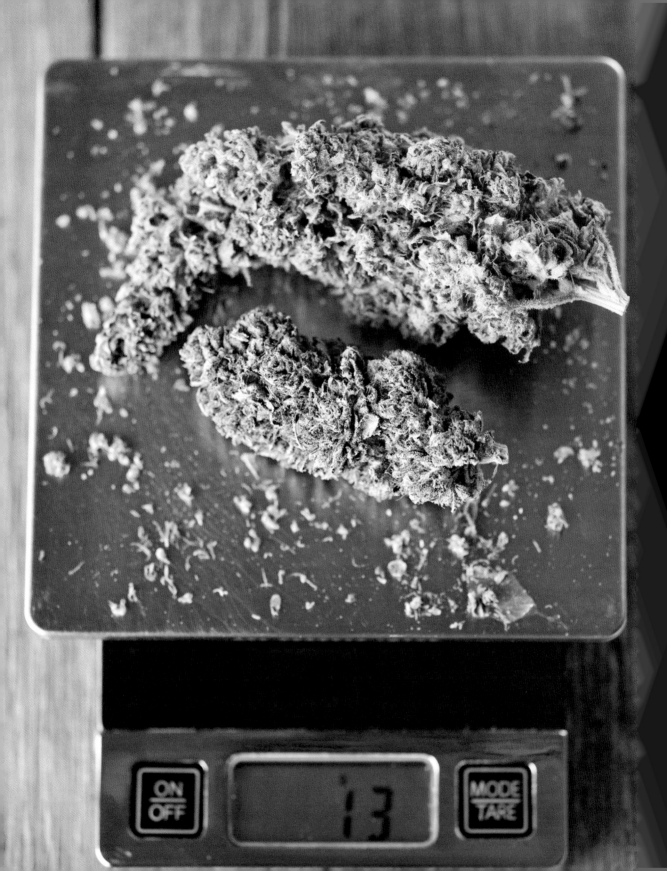

Equipment, Measurements, and Terms

Mise en place is a French phrase that means "put in place." It is used by chefs to refer to the way in which a cook organizes ingredients and equipment needed for a given recipe. Preparing in advance helps you stay focused while cooking. If you keep everything easily at hand, you won't ever have to worry that you have forgotten to add an ingredient. For recipes that must come together quickly, there will be no need to stop what you are doing to hunt down a specific ingredient, and no time wasted on measuring it. Mise en place makes life in the kitchen easier, your desserts more successful, and the art of baking sweeter.

The following is a list of equipment and terms useful to the home baker.

BAKING PANS Recipes for cookies were tested using an 11 x 15-inch baking sheet, but you can use whatever you have on hand. Make sure you follow directions for spacing the cookie dough. Baking sheets are also good to place under anything baked in a tart pan or a springform pan. Note that some recipes specify 10 x 15-inch sheets. An assortment of pan sizes are used in other recipes, including 10-inch springform, 10-inch Bundt, 10-inch tart, and 8- and 9-inch-square pans.

BOWLS   Have an assortment of sizes of stainless-steel and glass bowls available. Sizes used in the recipes range from a small, heatproof 6-ounce bowl (for making Hey Sugar!) up to 4- to 5-quart bowls.

CANDY THERMOMETER   There are only a few recipes in this book that require a candy thermometer, and to make these you can also use a laser temperature gun. You must have a laser temperature gun anyway; without it, you will not be able to determine the temperature of the cannabis you are decarboxylating. I mention the candy thermometer here only because you may already have one on hand, just sitting in a drawer and waiting for something to do.

For confections made at altitudes above sea level: Subtract 2 degrees Fahrenheit from the stated temperature for every 1,000 feet above sea level. For instance, if you live at 2,000 feet above sea level, the approximate conversion would be 4 degrees less than the stated candy temperature. In a recipe that calls for the candy to be brought to 240°F, you would boil it only to 236°F. Another example: If you live at 6,500 feet above sea level, the conversion factor would be 13 degrees less than the stated temperature (2 x 6 [thousand feet] + 1 degree for that extra 500 feet). If your recipe calls for 280°F, you would cook your candy to 267°F. As you can see, the higher the altitude, the more important it is to do this conversion. Even a few degrees can make a huge difference in the successful outcome of candy.

COFFEE FILTERS   You will need these for filtering the alcohol tincture for Hey Sugar! (See page 51 for the recipe.) Use unbleached filters.

COOKIE CUTTER   For the recipes in this book we used a 2-inch-round cookie cutter, but a glass with a 2-inch diameter also works. If the dough sticks, dip the rim of the glass in flour.

FOOD PROCESSOR   Use for prepping tart and pastry crusts, toppings, and fruit, and for chopping nuts and graham crackers.

GRINDER   This valuable little tool does just what the name says. When the buds are ground up, they have more surface area, which means increased potency. This maximizes the surface area of the plant matter that comes into contact with the product you are going to infuse, such as butter or coconut oil. A coffee grinder works well, or you can buy a grinder specifically made for grinding weed. They can be found in shops that sell pipes, papers, etc.

ICE CREAM MAKER   Any kind will work. Recipes for ice creams and sorbets were tested in both hand-crank and electric machines.

MASON JARS   These are needed for the Hey Sugar! recipe (see page 51) and also for making S'mores (see page 249).

MEASURING CUPS   You will need both liquid measuring cups and dry ingredient measuring cups. Dry ingredient measuring cups are meant to be filled right up to the top and then leveled off with a straight edge. Liquid measuring cups, generally made of glass or clear plastic, have a pouring spout. They are made to be filled to the measurements on the side, which are usually in both cup and ounce measurements.

MIXER   A handheld electric mixer was used to test most recipes in this book. If you don't own one, with a little bit of muscle, you can do the mixing by hand. If a stand mixer is necessary, it will say so in the recipe. If you own one, you can use it for most of the recipes.

OFFSET SPATULA   A thin, metal spatula where the blade is bent and sits about ½ inch below the handle. It allows you to smooth surfaces you can't reach with a regular flat spatula.

PAINT STRAINERS OR CHEESECLOTH   I find paint strainers easier to use than cheesecloth when pressing Buddha Budda (page 43) and Coconut Bliss (page 46). They don't tear easily and can be used over and over again. You can find them at hardware and paint stores. If you don't want to use these, or can't find them, use cheesecloth instead.

PARCHMENT PAPER OR SILICONE BAKING MATS   Depending on what I am making, I line all my baking sheets with one of these two items—unless the recipe calls for greasing the pan. In that case, a liner is unnecessary.

PASTRY BAGS AND TIPS   Although these are not strictly necessary, they give a professional finish when used to pipe frosting onto cupcakes and fillings into sandwich cookies.

PIE WEIGHTS   These are small, somewhat heavy objects used to weigh down a pie or tart crust that is being blind baked (baked without a filling); pie weights keep the crust nice and flat. They can be ceramic or stainless steel, or you can use uncooked rice or dried beans. The crust should be lined first with parchment paper or aluminum foil before the weights are added (make sure to cover the entire surface of the crust).

PYREX DISHES   Have an assortment of small to medium sizes available. You will need them for baking, for making Hey Sugar!, and for decarbing weed. Sizes are specified in the recipes.

RUBBER GLOVES   You'll need these when pressing Buddha Budda (page 43) and Coconut Bliss (page 46). The gloves protect your hands from the heat of the melted butter or coconut oil. Plus, having slippery butter or coconut oil all over your fingers is messy!

RULER   In order to cut cakes and brownies into even pieces, you will need a tape measure and also a sturdy metal ruler. Measure accurately!

SCALE   Get yourself a decent scale, one that weighs in both grams and ounces. Weight matters, particularly when it comes to dosing, and it's important to be accurate. Look for one with a tare button. To tare a scale, set an empty container on it and press the tare button. The scale will reset to zero, so when you add an ingredient to the container, the weight displayed will be just the weight of whatever you put *in* the container.

STRAINERS   For dusting powdered sugar over finished baked goods, and for pressing plant matter through when making Buddha Budda (page 43) and Coconut Bliss (page 46), I use good fine-mesh stainless-steel strainers in assorted sizes.

TEMPERATURE GUN, AKA LASER THERMOMETER   A noncontact infrared thermometer, which provides immediate feedback and reliable accuracy, is a must-have. It is the only way to test the temperature of the weed you will be decarbing (read more about decarbing on page 40). Available at most hardware stores.

TIMER   Digital or wind-up, it doesn't matter; the only thing that's important is that it works! You might think you'll remember to take those cookies out of the oven on time, but trust me, you probably won't.

TOOTHPICKS OR THIN WOODEN SKEWERS   I use these to test brownies and cakes for doneness.

TORCH   A small crème brûlée torch, found at most kitchen supply stores, will do the job.

WIRE COOLING RACKS Cooling racks are essential to create the perfect place for baked goods to cool down evenly and quickly. They allow air to circulate, preventing condensation and overbaking from residual heat from the pan.

Helpful Cooking Measurement Equivalents

1 tablespoon = 3 teaspoons

1/16 cup = 1 tablespoon

1/8 cup = 2 tablespoons

1/6 cup = 2 tablespoons + 2 teaspoons

1/4 cup = 4 tablespoons

1/3 cup = 5 tablespoons + 1 teaspoon

2/3 cup = 10 tablespoons + 2 teaspoons

3/8 cup = 6 tablespoons

1/2 cup = 8 tablespoons

2/3 cup = 10 tablespoons + 2 teaspoons

3/4 cup = 12 tablespoons

1 cup = 16 tablespoons

1 cup = 48 teaspoons

8 fluid ounces = 1 cup

1 pint = 2 cups

1 quart = 2 pints

4 cups = 1 quart

1 gallon = 4 quarts

16 ounces = 1 pound

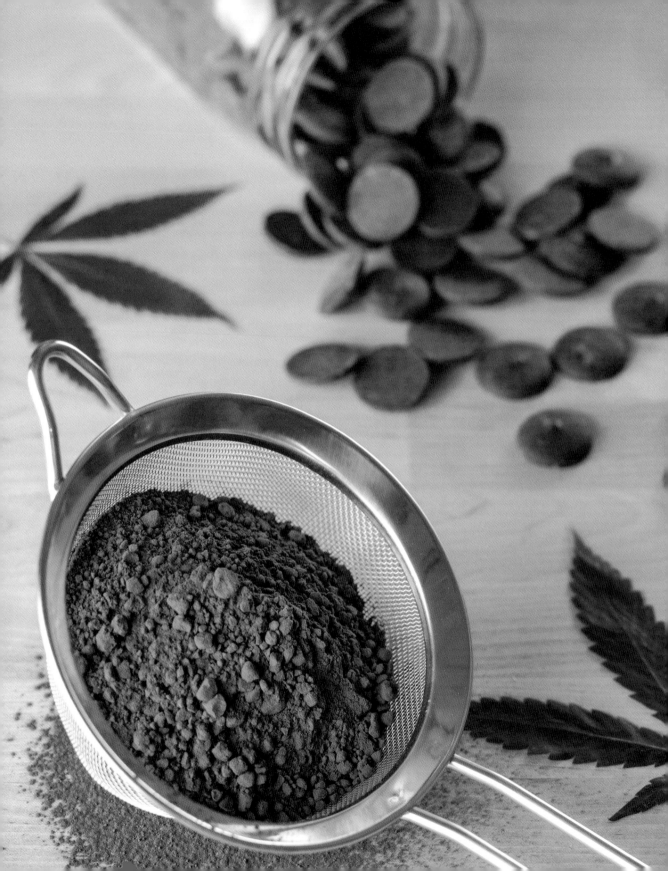

Ingredients

Almost all the ingredients used in these recipes (except for the cannabis) can be found in a good supermarket or natural foods store. Shop ethnic markets for specialty ingredients, such as rosewater or matcha powder.

Note: All ingredients should be brought to room temperature before baking, unless otherwise noted.

ARROWROOT POWDER   Extracted from the tuberous arrowroot plant, arrowroot powder, like cornstarch, is white, powdery, and used as a thickener. Unlike cornstarch, it contains no genetically modified organisms (GMOs).

BUDDHA BUDDA   Cannabis-infused butter (see recipe, page 43).

BUTTER   All recipes were tested with unsalted organic butter, unless otherwise noted.

CANNABIS   Try to find cannabis that was grown without pesticides. Most small home growers do not use them, but ask. Make sure it is completely dry before using.

CHOCOLATES   My favorites are Scharffen Berger, Divine, and Cocolove.

Bittersweet chocolate   Sweetened chocolate that contains at least 35 percent and up to 55 percent chocolate liquor (there is no alcohol in chocolate liquor).

Chocolate chips or chunks   These contain less cocoa butter than bar chocolate, which allows them to hold their shape when baked.

Cacao nibs   Small pieces of the roasted and hulled cacao bean. They are 100 percent pure cacao.

Cocoa powder   All recipes in this book that use cocoa were tested using either unsweetened Dutch-process or natural (also known as nonalkalized) cocoa powder. The difference between them is that Dutch-process cocoa gives a darker color and a more complex flavor, whereas natural cocoa powder tends to be fruitier tasting and lighter in color. Use whichever one you have on hand; for the recipes here it will not make a difference. To measure cocoa powder, first sift it to remove any lumps. Using a spoon, scoop the cocoa powder into the measuring cup without tapping the edge, then level off the excess cocoa powder with the back of a knife or an offset spatula.

High-percentage chocolate   Chocolate that contains 60 percent or higher chocolate liquor.

Milk chocolate   Sweetened chocolate with milk fat added. It contains a minimum of 10 percent cacao.

Semisweet chocolate   Sweetened chocolate that contains between 15 percent and 35 percent chocolate liquor.

Unsweetened chocolate   Chocolate liquor that has been cooled and molded into blocks to be used for baking. This is chocolate in its purest form, just cocoa solids and cocoa butter. It is 100 percent cacao.

White chocolate   This is a form of chocolate that contains no cacao. It is a blend of sugar, dry milk solids, milk fat, lecithin, and vanilla.

COCONUT BLISS   Cannabis-infused coconut oil (see recipe, page 46).

COCONUT OIL   We use certified organic virgin coconut oil.

COFFEE   For the most flavorful coffee or espresso flavor, use freshly ground beans.

DRIED FRUITS   These should be plump, moist, and full of flavor.

EGGS   All recipes were tested with large organic eggs, unless otherwise noted.

EXTRACTS   Always use pure extracts, never artificially flavored ones.

FLOUR   All recipes were tested using unbleached all-purpose flour (except for gluten-free recipes and the Hops to It Cupcakes, page 160, which uses cake flour) and were measured using the scoop-and-sweep method: Fluff up the flour in your canister with a whisk or fork and gently dip the cup into the flour to scoop it up, then sweep the top level with the back of a knife or an offset spatula.

Cake flour   Cake flour is a very finely ground flour that contains much less protein than all-purpose flour. It gives a softer and more tender texture to baked goods.

Gluten-free flour   Gluten-free recipes were tested with almond flour, rice flour, or Bob's Red Mill All-Purpose Baking Flour. To measure, use the scoop-and-sweep method (see above).

GANACHE   A mixture of chocolate and cream used for truffles, sauces, glazes, and cupcake and cake fillings.

MATCHA GREEN TEA POWDER   A premium green tea powder from Japan, used for drinking as tea or as an ingredient in recipes. It can be found in natural food stores or good tea shops.

ROSEWATER Produced by water distillation from rose flowers. Its delicate floral notes are an ideal complement to Middle Eastern, Indian, and Greek foods. It can be found in natural food stores or Middle Eastern specialty shops.

SPICES Use freshly ground spices. You can buy them in the bulk section of specialty stores or natural groceries; they are less expensive and fresher. Spices lose potency quickly, so buy only what you will use within the next few weeks.

VANILLA BEAN Vanilla beans are the fruit of an orchid. Be sure to purchase beans that are fresh, plump, and smooth. They are expensive, so store them in an airtight container and get every bit of the seeds out when scraping them. Here's how: Place the vanilla bean on a cutting board and split it in half lengthwise. Hold on to one end of the bean and firmly run a paring knife down the length of each half. After I've scraped the bean, I like to make vanilla sugar by placing the pod in a jar of sugar and letting it sit for two weeks. Keep adding pods as you use them.

VEGETABLE SHORTENING This is used for greasing pans and baking sheets.

SWEETENERS

BROWN SUGAR Dark and light brown sugar are refined sugar with molasses added to it. Both lend a butterscotchy, caramel flavor to the recipe. Brown sugar should be packed as it is measured.

GRANULATED WHITE Bleached and processed white sugar is a perfect sweetener; the flavor is neutral and doesn't clash with flavors of the ingredients in your baked goods.

HEY SUGAR! Cannabis-infused granulated white sugar (see recipe, page 51). When measuring, pack the measuring spoons or cups gently with your fingertips.

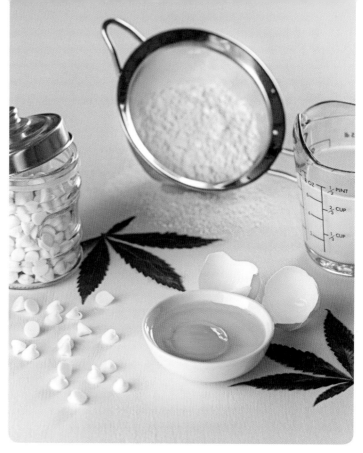

HONEY The flavor of honey varies with location and the type of flower the bees worked to produce the honey. These flavors include clover, mixed flower, orange blossom, and sage. Choose a flavor that pairs well with what you are baking. Before measuring, spray the inside of your measuring cup with cooking spray to make sure all of the honey comes out of the cup easily.

MOLASSES The juice extracted from sugarcane or sugar beets. Spray the inside of your measuring cup with cooking spray to make sure all of the molasses comes out of the cup easily.

POWDERED SUGAR Also known as confectioners' sugar or icing sugar. It is made by milling granulated sugar.

RAW SUGAR Semirefined sugar with some molasses left in it.

Infusions

BUDDHA BUDDA · *43*

COCONUT BLISS · *46*

A WORD ABOUT SWEET LEAF · *49*

HEY SUGAR! · *51*

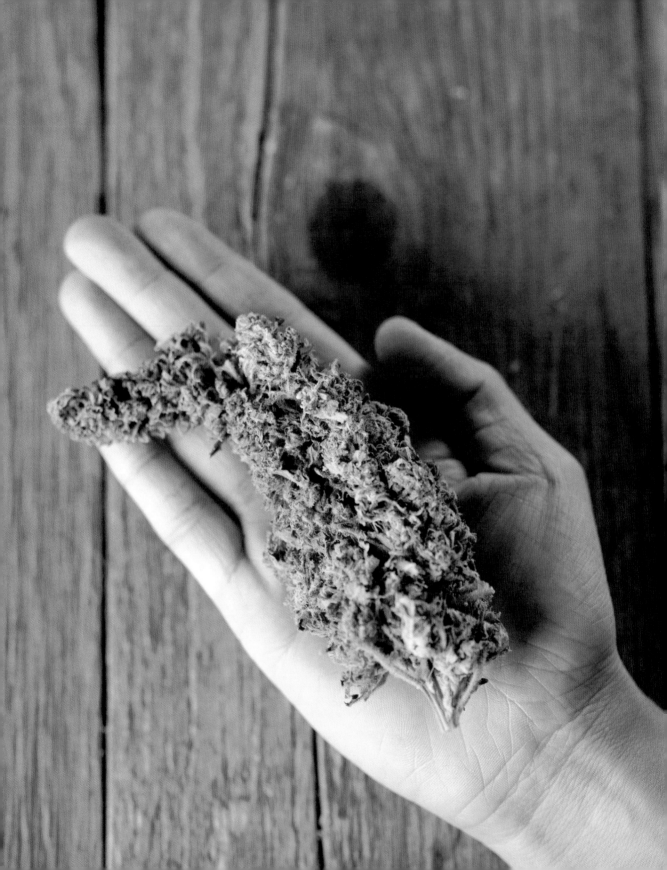

*C*annabis-infused butter (Buddha Budda), coconut oil (Coconut Bliss), and sugar (Hey Sugar!) are the basis for every recipe in this cookbook. Please read this section carefully.

Infused edible products are a drug—not a food—and they can be used safely and effectively by exercising caution and starting with low levels of THC. But I want you to read this section three times before you go anywhere near your kitchen!

This Will Feel Different from Smoking

Edibles are not the same as smoked or vaporized cannabis. Each form has its own characteristic chemistry, dosing, onset, and duration; the slow start and extended duration of oral cannabis can come as a surprise to those familiar only with smoking or vaporizing. Even frequent smokers can overdo it when ingesting. So if you think your weed-smoking tolerance has prepped you for higher-milligram usage in edibles, think again. While no one has died from an overdose of cannabis, overdosing can be extremely distressing, resulting in paranoia, disorientation, out-of-body experience, nausea, vomiting, pounding heart, anxiety, and hallucinations.

Learn Your Tolerance

Don't start with the higher doses of THC. Please be cautious, especially if you are a rookie. Learn your tolerance. Don't listen to what anyone else says about their experience. Effects can vary dramatically, depending on individual body chemistry, the type and potency of the product, and how much you have consumed. What was too little to get someone else high might cause you to overdose. Overdosing means that you have taken more than the normal or recommended amount. As already mentioned, an overdose of cannabis is not fatal, but it can be mighty unpleasant.

I thought a lot about dosing when I started this cookbook. Did I want the confections to be super-dosed, as most of the Colorado market demands? Or did I want you guys to be able to eat a whole cookie, brownie, or slice of a tart? It seems silly to restrict you to a little piece of a cookie because the whole would be too strong, so I decided to go with the latter option. You can always have seconds, but *only after* you've waited to see how you feel after the first serving. Read more below.

Be Patient

I've said it before here, and don't worry, I'll say it again, because this is important. Listen up: When you *smoke* marijuana, you receive only a small amount of the cannabinoids with each hit, and you feel it immediately; but when you ingest infused treats, the cannabinoids are released in waves as they are processed by the digestive system.

It takes between *30 and 120 minutes* to feel the first effects. It might be another three hours before the full potency kicks in, and then it's another three to six hours before you're back to baseline. So WAIT before you take more. Be patient. Learn how your metabolism works with infused treats. And when testing the edible waters, make sure you have ample time to do so. Don't have a High-End Celestial Cookie (page 107) four hours before a job interview.

Don't Bake Stoned

Another important point: When experimenting with new edibles, always start sober. This means *do not bake stoned, and do not eat an edible if you are already stoned*. Starting sober is the only way to learn what your tolerance level is. Here in Colorado there is a saying: "Start low. Go slow." Please keep that in mind.

Mark Edibles Clearly

Mark whatever you are storing your edibles in with a clear warning, so that people will know exactly what they're getting. Sweets left out are always a temptation, and an unsuspecting sweet-stealer might eat two or three cookies and then be sidelined for hours. Make sure everyone in the home understands that these are infused desserts. These treats are a drug, and people need to know what they are before popping them into their mouths.

Keep Track of Dosing

Know the approximate number of milligrams of THC in each treat. Dosage is important. Some people may only be able to handle a 10-milligram brownie—you don't want them eating a 50-milligram brownie.

KEEP OUT OF REACH OF CHILDREN

ALWAYS!

Decarboxylation

Cooking with THC is not just about adding cannabis to butter. You want to make sure you get the most out of your weed—you spent good money to buy it!

THC-A, also known as Tetrahydrocannabinolic acid, is non-psychoactive—it is unactivated THC, the biosynthetic precursor to THC (Delta-9-tetrahydrocannabinol, also known as Δ-9 THC). THC is what produces the psychoactive effect of feeling "high." What you need to do is convert *un*activated THC-A into *activated* THC. This is accomplished through a process called decarboxylation—the removal of CO_2.

Unactivated THC-A still has many therapeutic benefits. For instance, it helps with chronic immune system disorders; it also has anti-inflammatory properties, is antiproliferative (meaning that it inhibits the growth of cancer cells), and it can help control muscle spasms. But as long as the extra CO_2 of THC-A is attached to the THC, potency is suppressed.

Not all strains of cannabis are created equal. The levels of THC in baked goods are approximate, depending on the quality of the cannabis, but also on how well you have decarboxylated. When I first started Sweet Mary Jane, I didn't decarb, because I didn't know about the process. I'd send my infused butter, sugar, or coconut oil to the lab, and the report would come back indicating that a high percentage of THC-A had not been activated. It wasn't turning into THC! So while decarbing is a little time consuming, it is a must.

Here's the deal: I am going to show you how to make treats using infusions of THC in butter, coconut oil, and sugar that start with a dose as low as about 6.25 milligrams per serving and go up to about 50 milligrams per serving. (Just so you know, 50 milligrams is a lot of THC!) Without the benefit of lab testing, you won't know your exact cannabinoid content, but we can get fairly close to these levels.

The following recipes give amounts needed to make a range of doses, but the first few times you make Buddha Budda (cannabis-infused butter), Coconut Bliss (cannabis-infused coconut oil), and Hey Sugar! (cannabis-infused sugar), you should aim for the lowest dose.

To get the milligrams of THC per serving: Take the total milligrams of THC that you've added to your recipe and divide by the number of servings the recipe yields. (All the recipes can be easily doubled.)

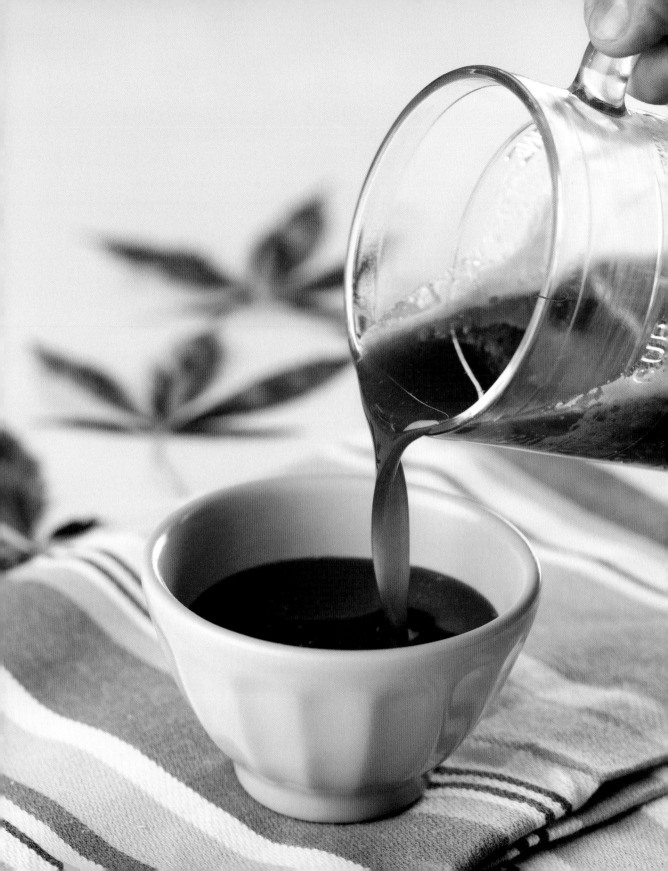

Buddha Budda

Buddha Budda can be spread on toast or muffins, or melted on waffles or pancakes; basically, you can use it any place you would normally use butter. It can also be substituted for butter in any of your favorite recipes.

As you will see in the recipes below, the amount of bud used determines the level of THC in finished desserts, with three levels of dosing.

Yield for each of the following recipes is ½ cup, or 8 tablespoons, of Buddha Budda.

LEVEL 1

1½ grams cannabis buds, ground or finely crushed
½ cup (8 tablespoons/1 stick) unsalted butter

Yield: about 150 mg THC total

1 tablespoon = about 18.75 mg THC

12 edibles: about 12.5 mg THC each

18 edibles: about 8.3 mg THC each

LEVEL 2

3 grams cannabis buds, ground or finely crushed
½ cup (8 tablespoons/1 stick) unsalted butter

Yield: about 300 mg THC total

1 tablespoon = about 37.5 mg THC

12 edibles: about 25 mg THC each

18 edibles: about 16.6 mg THC each

LEVEL 3 🌿 🌿 🌿

6 grams cannabis buds, ground or finely crushed
½ cup (8 tablespoons/1 stick) unsalted butter

Yield: about 600 mg THC total

1 tablespoon = about 75 mg THC

12 edibles: about 50 mg THC total

18 edibles: about 33.3 mg THC total

Infusion Tools
Digital temperature gun (it's the only way to test the temperature of the weed)
Decent digital scale that weighs both grams and ounces
Paint-straining bags or cheesecloth
Large bowl
Strainer
Rubber gloves

1. Decarboxylate the cannabis: Preheat the oven to 250°F. Put the cannabis in a small, heat-proof baking dish and place in the oven. After 15 to 20 minutes, check the temperature of the cannabis with your digital temperature gun; once it has reached 250°F, let it bake for 30 minutes, checking the temperature frequently. (In addition to decarboxylating, you are removing any moisture left in the plant material.) If it goes over the correct temperature for too long, it will burn, the THC may convert into CBN, and you will lose potency. (See the chart on page 279 in Appendix A for information about cannabinoids.) Remove from the oven and set aside to cool. If not using immediately, store the cannabis in an airtight container in a dark place for up to 2 months.

2. Melt the butter in a small saucepan over medium-low heat. Add the decarbed weed and bring the temperature of the butter up to 190°F. Cook for 30 minutes, using the digital temperature gun to check the temperature

of the butter frequently and make sure it does not go over 200°F. DO NOT LEAVE UNATTENDED! (If by chance it does go over 200°F for a few minutes, don't worry, it isn't ruined. The THC is still in there. But excessive heating causes degradation of THC and may convert it to CBN, one of the cannabinoids responsible for the sedative effects of cannabis, or result in vaporization of the compounds. Inadequate heating isn't good either, as it causes the majority of the cannabinoids to remain in their acid form and thus unactivated. The density of the product, and the time and temperature of the oven, can also prevent some conversion, which results in unactivated cannabinoids. Adding the decarbed cannabis to the butter or coconut oil and heating it again ensures a better conversion.) Mostly, you want to keep everything at a simmer, not a boil. Just turn down the heat and watch it.

3. Take the saucepan off the heat and let it sit for 10 minutes.

4. It's now time to press. Place a strainer over a large bowl. Place a paint strainer or cheesecloth into the strainer, folding down the sides over the outside. Spoon the infused butter into it. Using a large spoon or potato masher, press as much as you can through the cloth. Then, using your hands (rubber gloves help here!), squeeze the bag. Press out as much of the precious liquid as you can. Measure the amount you have left. Normally, there is about a 25 percent loss; this is not a loss of THC. Make up the difference with regular melted butter.

5. Buddha Budda can be stored in an airtight container for up to 8 weeks in the refrigerator. It also freezes well, so make more if you have the bud and freeze the extra batch in an airtight container for up to 6 months.

Coconut Bliss

Coconut Bliss can be used anywhere you would use coconut oil. The oil can also be consumed on its own; many patients medicate by taking a spoonful every day (the size of the spoon determines the dosage). A rich source of saturated fats, coconut oil contains a lot of medium-chain triglycerides, which are metabolized differently than longer-chain triglycerides, and can have therapeutic effects on different disorders. These health benefits are attributed to the antimicrobial, antioxidant, antifungal, antibacterial, and soothing properties of the oil's lauric acid, capric acid, and caprylic acid. (See Appendix A, page 279, for more information.)

As you will see in the recipes below, the amount of bud used determines the level of THC in finished desserts, with three levels of dosing.

Yield for each of the following recipes is ½ cup, or 8 tablespoons, of Coconut Bliss.

LEVEL 1

1½ grams cannabis buds, ground or finely crushed
½ cup (8 tablespoons) coconut oil

Yield: about 150 mg THC total

1 tablespoon = about 18.75 mg THC

12 edibles: about 12.5 mg THC each

18 edibles: about 8.3 mg THC each

LEVEL 2

3 grams cannabis buds, ground or finely crushed
½ cup (8 tablespoons) coconut oil

Yield: about 300 mg THC total

1 tablespoon = about 37.5 mg THC

12 edibles: about 25 mg THC each

18 edibles: about 16.6 mg THC each

LEVEL 3 ⧜ ⧜ ⧜

6 grams cannabis buds, ground or finely crushed
½ cup (8 tablespoons) coconut oil

Yield: about 600 mg THC total

1 tablespoon = about 75 mg THC

12 edibles: about 50 mg THC each

18 edibles: about 33.3 mg THC each

Infusion Tools
Digital temperature gun (it's the only way to test the temperature of the weed)
Decent digital scale that weighs both grams and ounces
Paint-straining bags or cheesecloth
Large bowl
Strainer
Rubber gloves

1. Decarboxylate the cannabis: Preheat the oven to 250°F. Put the cannabis in a small, heat-proof baking dish and place in the oven. After 15 to 20 minutes, check the temperature of the cannabis with your digital temperature gun; once it has reached 250°F, let it bake for 30 minutes, checking the temperature frequently. (In addition to decarboxylating, you are removing any moisture left in the plant material.) If it goes over the correct temperature for too long, it will burn, the THC may convert into CBN, and you will lose potency. (See the chart on page 279 in Appendix A for information about cannabinoids.) Remove from the oven and set aside to cool. If not using immediately, store the cannabis in an airtight container in a dark place for up to 2 months.

2. Melt the coconut oil in a small saucepan over medium-low heat. Add the

decarbed weed and bring the temperature of the butter up to 190°F. Cook for 30 minutes, using the digital temperature gun to check the temperature of the butter frequently and make sure it does not go over 200°F. DO NOT LEAVE UNATTENDED! (If by chance it does go over 200°F for a few minutes, don't worry, it isn't ruined. The THC is still in there. But excessive heating causes degradation of THC and may convert it to CBN, one of the cannabinoids responsible for the sedative effects of cannabis, or result in vaporization of the compounds. Inadequate heating isn't good either, as it causes the majority of the cannabinoids to remain in their acid form and thus unactivated. The density of the product, and the time and temperature of the oven, can also prevent some conversion, which results in unactivated cannabinoids. Adding the decarbed cannabis to the butter or coconut oil and heating it again ensures a better conversion.) Mostly, you want to keep everything at a simmer, not a boil. Just turn down the heat and watch it.

3. Take the saucepan off the heat and let it sit for 10 minutes.

4. It's now time to press. Place a strainer over a large bowl. Place a paint strainer or cheesecloth into the strainer, folding down the sides over the outside. Spoon the infused coconut oil into it. Using a large spoon or potato masher, press as much as you can through the cloth. Then, using your hands (rubber gloves help here!), squeeze the bag. Press out as much of the precious liquid as you can. Measure the amount you have left. Normally, there is about a 25 percent loss; this is not a loss of THC. Make up the difference with regular coconut oil.

5. Coconut Bliss can be stored in an airtight container in the refrigerator for up to 8 weeks. It also freezes well, so make more if you have the bud and freeze the extra batch in an airtight container for up to 6 months.

A Word About Sweet Leaf

Sweet leaf is a term that refers to the plant matter trimmed from around the mature buds of the cannabis plant. These leaves grow close to the flower tops, nearest to the plant's resin—they look as if they've been dusted with sugar—and therefore contain a high concentration of medicinal compounds. If you have access to good-quality sweet leaf, use it! Make sure it's dry before beginning decarboxylation. Follow the directions for making Buddha Budda or Coconut Bliss.

LEVEL 1 🌿

9 grams sweet leaf, ground or finely crushed
2 cups unsalted butter or coconut oil

> *Yield: 48 pieces at about 12.5 mg THC each*

LEVEL 2 🌿 🌿

18 grams sweet leaf, ground or finely crushed
2 cups unsalted butter or coconut oil

> *Yield: 48 pieces at about 25 mg THC each*

LEVEL 3 🌿 🌿 🌿

36 grams sweet leaf, ground or finely crushed
2 cups unsalted butter or coconut oil

> *Yield: 48 pieces at about 50 mg THC each*

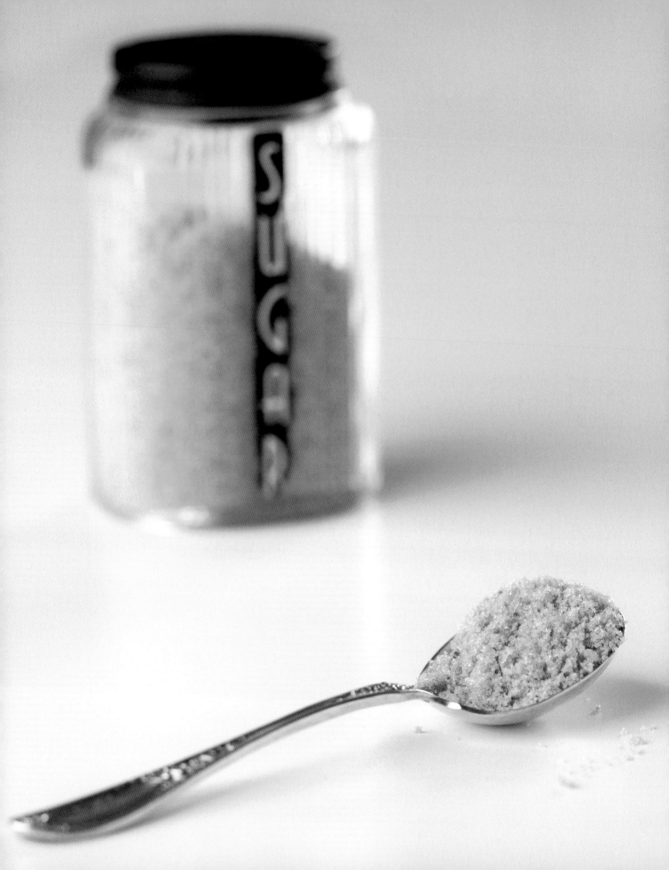

Hey Sugar!

At Sweet Mary Jane, for the first few years we infused all our baked goods with Buddha Budda or Coconut Bliss. But, eventually, I wanted to try another technique. After some experimenting, I came up with the idea of infusing sugar. It turned out to be a genuine innovation. The beauty of infused sugar is that there is much less cannabis flavor and color in the finished product. Many of the confections we sell use Hey Sugar!. We also sell packages of it for people to use to sweeten their coffee or tea, or to bake with at home.

Use the highest-proof alcohol you can find. If you have access to Everclear, use that. Otherwise, Bacardi 151 rum will do the trick (if not quite as well).

Hey Sugar! can be dropped into any hot drink. If you want to add it to a cold drink, heat a small portion of the liquid, add the Hey Sugar!, stir to dissolve, and then add it to your drink. It can also be substituted for sugar in any of your favorite recipes.

As you will see in the following recipes, the amount of bud used determines the level of THC in the finished desserts, with three levels of dosing.

Yield for each of the following recipes is ¼ cup of Hey Sugar!.

LEVEL 1

1½ grams cannabis buds, ground or finely crushed
¼ cup granulated sugar

Yield: about 150 mg THC total

1 teaspoon = about 12.5 mg THC

LEVEL 2 ✿ ✿

3 grams cannabis buds, ground or finely crushed
¼ cup granulated sugar

> *Yield: about 300 mg THC total*
>
> *1 teaspoon = about 25 mg THC*

LEVEL 3 ✿ ✿ ✿

6 grams cannabis buds, ground or finely crushed
¼ cup granulated sugar

> *Yield: about 600 mg THC total*
>
> *1 teaspoon = about 50 mg THC*

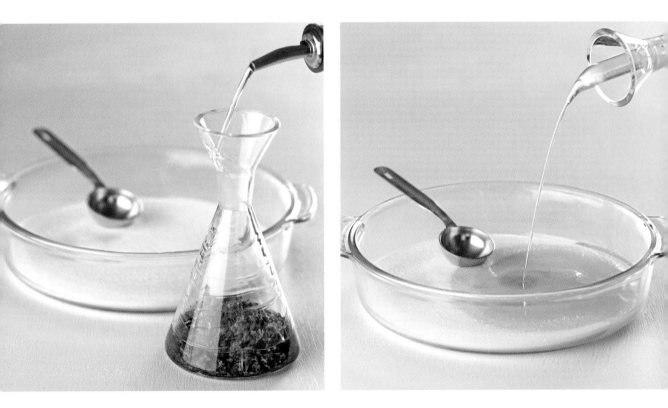

2 mason jars
Funnel
Coffee filter
Small heat-proof baking dish
Heat-proof glass pie dish
High-proof alcohol: Everclear works best—however,
   not every state sells it; if you can't purchase it, use Bacardi 151 rum

1. Decarboxylate the cannabis: Preheat the oven to 250°F. Put the cannabis in a small, heat-proof baking dish and place in the oven. After 15 to 20 minutes, check the temperature of the cannabis with your digital temperature gun; once it has reached 250°F, let it bake for 30 minutes, checking the temperature frequently. (In addition to decarboxylating, you are removing any moisture left in the plant material.) If it goes over the correct temperature for too long, it will burn, the THC may convert into CBN, and you will lose potency. (See the chart on page 279 in Appendix A for information about cannabinoids.) If not using immediately, store the cannabis in an airtight container in a dark place for up to 2 months.

2. Remove the baking dish from the oven and reduce the oven temperature to 200°F. Transfer the cannabis to a mason jar. Pour in just enough alcohol to cover it, and seal the jar. Shake the jar every 3 to 5 minutes for 20 minutes, then open the lid.

3. Line a strainer with a coffee filter and place it over a bowl. Pour the alcohol solution through the coffee filter to strain off the plant matter. Gently press with the back of a spoon or your fingertips, being careful not to break the filter.

4. Place the sugar in a heat-proof glass pie dish. Add the strained alcohol solution to the sugar and bake for 30 to 60 minutes, stirring well every

10 minutes, until all the liquid has evaporated and the sugar is evenly colored. (The color can range from light to dark amber.)

5. Store in an airtight container in a cool, dark place. There is no need to refrigerate. Hey Sugar! is good for 1 year.

How to Calculate Doses

The level of THC in cannabis, and therefore the potency of the cannabis, is not always consistent. The way in which the plant is grown, which nutrients are used, how it is cured, and differences in the chemical composition of cannabis varieties all affect the amount of THC produced. Below, I've outlined a basic way to calculate potency of your baked goods, but since the level of THC in your cannabis may differ from what I've listed, be extra cautious and always start at the lowest infusion level.

To find out the number of milligrams of THC per serving and per recipe, please refer to Infusions (pages 43 to 53). For your selected level of infusion, multiply the number of tablespoons of the infusion you are using in your recipe by the milligrams of THC per tablespoon given in the Infusions chapter. The resulting number is your total dosage for the full recipe. Divide this number by the total number of servings in the recipe to get your dose per serving.

For example, if you're making the Alice bars (page 58) at the lowest dosing level:

Infusion included in recipe = 8 tablespoons
THC per tablespoon = 18.75 mg THC
Number of servings = 12 servings

Infusion in recipe (½ cup = 8 tablespoons)

× THC per tablespoon (18.75 mg THC)

= Total THC in recipe (150 mg THC)

÷ Servings per recipe (12 servings)

= THC per serving (12.5 mg THC per serving)

Make sure to calculate the THC per recipe and per serving anytime you bake with cannabis, to keep control of your dosing.

Brownies and Bars

ALICE · *58*

ALEX'S MINT MADNESS · *60*

GOOD DAY SUNSHINE · *63*

LEMON LOVE BARS · *67*

MERCIFUL · *69*

OMG! BROWNIE CHEESECAKE BARS · *73*

RASPBERRY JAM SESSION · *77*

SMASHING PUMPKIN BARS · *81*

WALNUT FANTASY · *83*

MARK T'S RAW BAR YOGI TREATS · *85*

Alice

Alice in Wonderland? Alice B. Toklas? Alice Waters? Take your pick—this blond bombshell has all good things to offer—sweet, enchanting, always up for something new. Substitute any dried fruit, or leave the fruit out and add nuts, or do both. Same goes for the white chocolate. Try milk chocolate instead, dark chocolate, or butterscotch chips. It's all good.

Makes 12 bars

THC per serving: Please see page 54 to calculate.

Vegetable shortening, for greasing the pan
½ cup Buddha Budda (page 43), melted
1 cup light brown sugar
1 large egg
1 teaspoon pure vanilla extract
¼ teaspoon salt
1 cup all-purpose flour
½ cup dried cranberries
½ cup white chocolate chips

1. Preheat the oven to 350°F. Grease a 9 x 9-inch baking pan with vegetable shortening.

2. In a large bowl using an electric mixer, beat the melted Buddha Budda with the sugar on medium speed until smooth. Beat in the egg and then the vanilla. With the mixer on low, add the salt and flour. Fold in the cranberries and white chocolate chips.

3. Pour the batter into the prepared pan. Bake for 20 to 25 minutes, or until a toothpick inserted into the center comes out with a few moist crumbs

clinging to it. Do not overbake; a gooey center works here. Let cool completely before cutting into 12 equal-size bars. Wrap tightly in aluminum foil and store in the refrigerator for up to 1 week, or in the freezer for up to 3 months.

Alex's Mint Madness

....

Alex Ivers, one of *Sweet Mary Jane's* top bakers, came up with this recipe, a cool mint filling sandwiched between a fudgy brownie base and a milk chocolate glaze. It's based on a brownie he fondly remembers from his childhood, and with a few tweaks, it's become a treat that Sweet Mary Jane fans adore.

Makes 12 brownies

THC per serving: Please see page 54 to calculate.

Vegetable shortening, for greasing the foil

Brownie Layer

½ cup Buddha Budda (page 43), slightly softened
1 cup granulated sugar
1 (16-ounce) can chocolate syrup
1 teaspoon pure vanilla extract
4 large eggs
1 cup all-purpose flour
⅛ teaspoon salt

Filling

½ cup (8 tablespoons/1 stick) unsalted butter
2 cups powdered sugar
2 tablespoons whole milk
1½ teaspoons peppermint extract
10 to 12 drops green food coloring

Milk Chocolate Glaze

11.5 ounces milk chocolate chips
3 tablespoons Buddha Budda (page 43)
6 tablespoons (¾ stick) unsalted butter

1. Preheat the oven to 350°F. Line an 11 x 15-inch baking pan with foil, pressing it into the corners and letting about 3 inches hang over two opposite sides of the pan. Grease the foil with vegetable shortening.

2. Prepare the brownie layer: In a large bowl using an electric mixer, cream together the Buddha Budda and granulated sugar on medium speed until light and fluffy. Add the chocolate syrup and vanilla. Add the eggs one at a time until well combined. Reduce the mixer speed to low and add the flour and salt; mix until smooth. Pour the batter into the prepared pan and bake for 20 minutes, or until a toothpick inserted into the center comes out with a few moist crumbs clinging to it. Set the pan on a wire rack to cool while you prepare the filling.

3. Prepare the filling: In a large bowl using an electric mixer, cream together the butter and powdered sugar on medium speed. Add the milk and mix until the filling is spreadable. Beat in the peppermint extract and food coloring. Spread the filling over the baked brownie layer, cover, and refrigerate until the filling is firm, 30 to 45 minutes.

4. Prepare the chocolate glaze: Combine the chocolate chips, Buddha Budda, and butter in a small saucepan over low heat. Stir the mixture until the chips are melted and smooth. Pour the glaze over the chilled brownies, tilting the pan so that the glaze covers the entire surface. Refrigerate until the glaze has hardened, 30 to 45 minutes.

5. Using the overhanging foil, lift the brownie block out of the pan and place on a cutting board. Cut into 12 equal-size bars. Wrap tightly in aluminum foil and store in the refrigerator for up to 1 week, or in the freezer for up to 3 months.

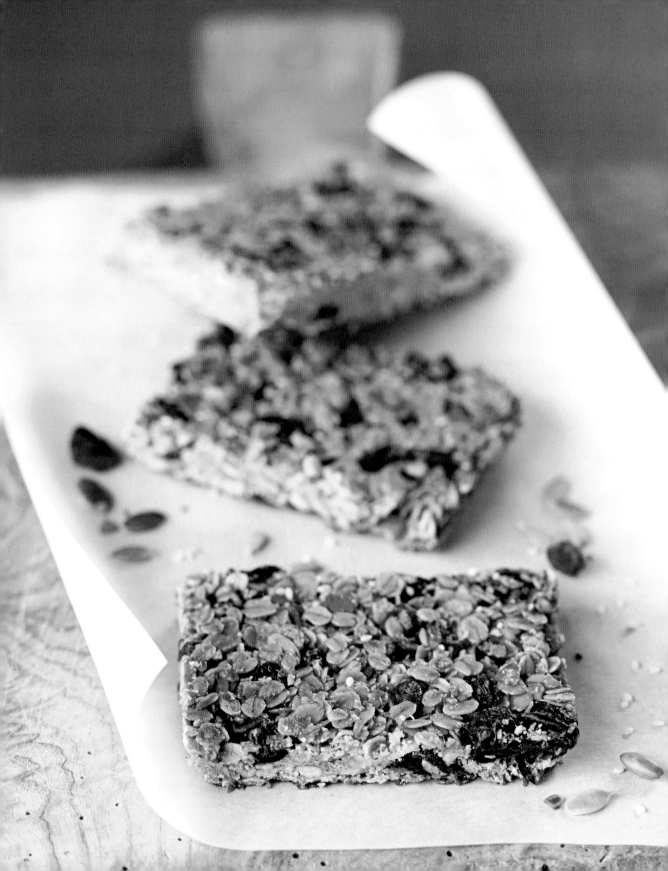

Good Day Sunshine

Maple-y sweet goodness all wrapped up in a healthy bar, chockablock with nuts, fruits, and seeds. These are tricky to get out of the pan, so carefully follow the instructions for preparing the pan. If you are gluten-intolerant, be sure the oats are labeled gluten-free. Make these vegan by using Coconut Bliss rather than Buddha Budda.

Makes 9 bars

THC per serving: Please see page 54 to calculate.

Vegetable shortening, for greasing the pan
¼ cup shredded unsweetened coconut
2 cups old-fashioned rolled oats
½ cup mixed seeds, such as hemp, sunflower, pumpkin, flax, chia, and sesame
1½ cups mixed dried fruit, such as raisins, cherries, blueberries, and cranberries
2 teaspoons ground cinnamon
6 tablespoons Buddha Budda (page 43) or Coconut Bliss (page 46)
½ cup honey
⅓ cup firmly packed dark brown sugar
⅓ cup pure maple syrup
¼ teaspoon salt
2 tablespoons pure vanilla extract

1. Preheat the oven to 350°F. Grease a 9 x 9-inch baking pan with vegetable shortening and line it with foil, pressing it into the corners and letting about 4 inches hang over two opposite sides of the pan. Grease the foil and dust the bottom and sides with shredded coconut. Sprinkle any remaining coconut over the bottom of the baking pan.

2. Spread the oats and seeds evenly on a rimmed baking sheet and toast in the oven just until golden and fragrant, 6 to 8 minutes.

3. In a large bowl, toss together the toasted oats and seeds, dried fruit, and cinnamon. Set aside.

4. In a saucepan, combine the Buddha Budda, honey, brown sugar, maple syrup, and salt. Set over medium heat and stir until smooth and hot. Remove from the heat and stir in the vanilla. Pour the hot sugar mixture into the oat mixture and stir until well combined. Pour the batter into the prepared pan, pressing it into the pan evenly with an offset spatula.

5. Bake until lightly browned, 25 to 30 minutes. Transfer the pan to a wire rack and let cool completely.

6. Using the overhanging foil, gently lift out of the pan and place on a cutting board. Refrigerate for 1 hour. Cut into 9 equal-size bars. Wrap tightly in aluminum foil and store in the refrigerator for up to 2 weeks, or in the freezer for up to 3 months.

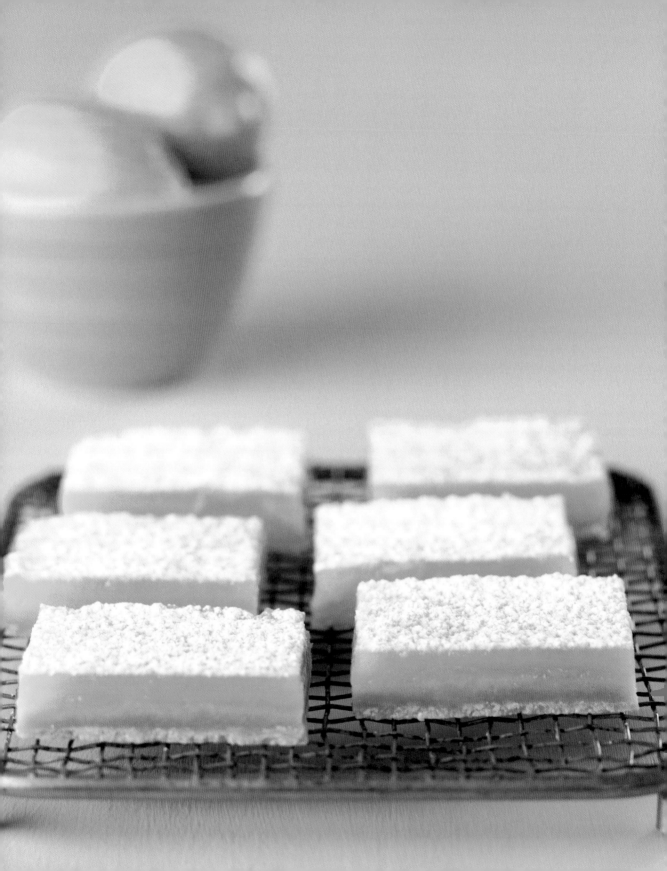

Lemon Love Bars

....

These sunny lemon bars might just put a spring in your step. The key ingredient is freshly squeezed lemon juice. I top a shortbread pastry crust with a zingy filling, and dust the whole thing with a snowy sprinkling of powdered sugar. The flavor is tangy and not too sweet.

Makes 12 bars

THC per serving: Please see page 54 to calculate.

Vegetable shortening, for greasing the pan

Crust
1½ cups all-purpose flour
⅓ cup granulated sugar
¼ teaspoon salt
1 tablespoon lemon zest
½ cup Buddha Budda (page 43), cut into pieces and chilled

Filling
4 large eggs
1⅓ cups granulated sugar
1 cup fresh lemon juice

Powdered sugar, for dusting

1. Preheat the oven to 350°F. Grease a 9 x 9-inch baking pan with vegetable shortening and line it with foil, pressing it into the corners and letting about 3 inches hang over two opposite sides of the pan.

2. Prepare the crust: In the bowl of a food processor, combine the flour, granulated sugar, salt, and lemon zest and pulse to combine. Add the Buddha Budda and pulse in short bursts until the mixture forms coarse, sandy

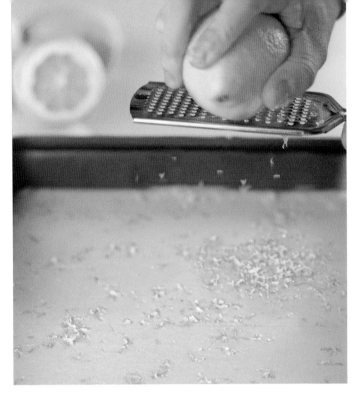

crumbs. Transfer the dough to the prepared pan and press it into an even layer. Place in the freezer for 15 minutes. (Set the food processor bowl aside—you're going to use it again.)

3. Remove the pan from the freezer and bake for 15 to 18 minutes, until the crust is just lightly golden brown around the edges. Leave the oven on.

4. While the crust is baking, prepare the filling: In the food processor bowl, combine the eggs, granulated sugar, and lemon juice and pulse to combine well.

5. Pour the filling over the hot crust and return the pan to the oven for about 20 minutes more, or until the filling is just set. Transfer to a wire rack. Put 2 to 3 tablespoons powdered sugar in a strainer and dust the top.

6. When the bars are completely cooled, refrigerate for at least 1 hour before cutting into 12 equal-size bars. Dust each bar with another sprinkling of powdered sugar. Wrap tightly in aluminum foil and store in the refrigerator for up to 1 week, or in the freezer for up to 3 months.

Merciful

....

A pot brownie is the quintessential infused treat, and Merciful was one of the first brownies on the Sweet Mary Jane menu. Maybe, when weed became legal here, people were looking for an item they already knew, but I have found that everyone gravitates to what tastes best. Merciful is a delicious brownie made with four different kinds of chocolate, and it is still one of our top sellers.

Makes 18 brownies

THC per serving: Please see page 54 to calculate.

Vegetable shortening, for greasing the pan
¾ cup Buddha Budda (page 43)
¼ cup (4 tablespoons/½ stick) unsalted butter
10 ounces semisweet chocolate
4 ounces unsweetened chocolate
6 tablespoons unsweetened cocoa powder
6 large eggs
2½ cups sugar
1 teaspoon salt
1 tablespoon pure vanilla extract
2 cups all-purpose flour

Drizzle
½ cup white chocolate chips
¼ teaspoon vegetable shortening

1. Preheat the oven to 350°F. Grease a 10 x 15-inch baking pan.

2. In a small saucepan, melt the Buddha Budda and butter together over low heat. Add the semisweet and unsweetened chocolates and cook, stirring, until the chocolates have melted. Whisk in the cocoa powder and remove from the heat.

3. In a medium bowl, whisk together the eggs, sugar, salt, and vanilla until well combined. Add the chocolate mixture and whisk well. Fold in the flour.

4. Pour the batter into the prepared pan. Bake for 18 to 20 minutes, or until a toothpick inserted into the center comes out with a few moist crumbs clinging to it. Let cool completely before cutting into 18 equal-size bars.

5. Prepare the drizzle: In the top section of a double boiler, melt the white chocolate and the shortening over simmering water. Stir continuously until the chocolate has melted, being careful not to get any water into the chocolate or it will seize (see Note).

6. Dip a fork into the melted chocolate and drizzle it over the tops of the brownies. Let the chocolate set. Wrap tightly in aluminum foil and store in the refrigerator for up to 1 week, or in the freezer for up to 3 months.

Note: Chocolate should melt into a smooth, satiny pool, but it's temperamental and will not tolerate moisture. If even the tiniest bit of condensation drips down the inside of a pan, or if steam escapes from the bottom of the double boiler, the chocolate will react badly, becoming a grainy mess; this is known as "seizing."

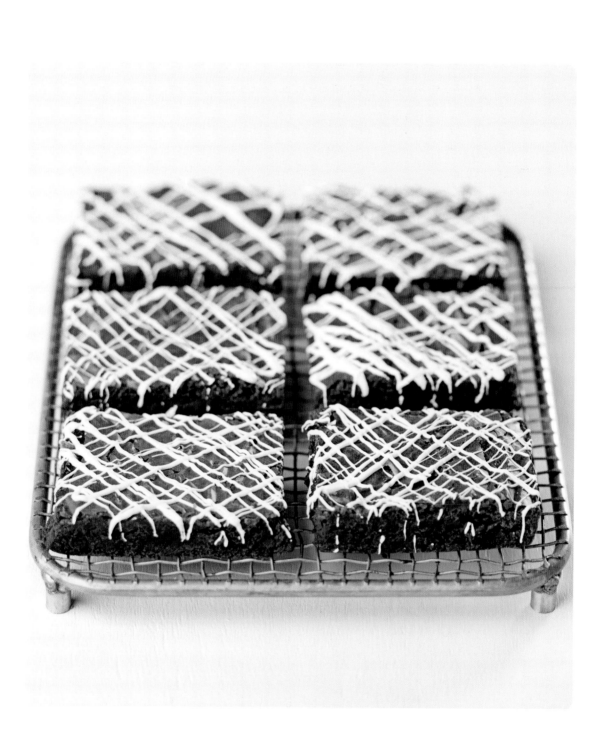

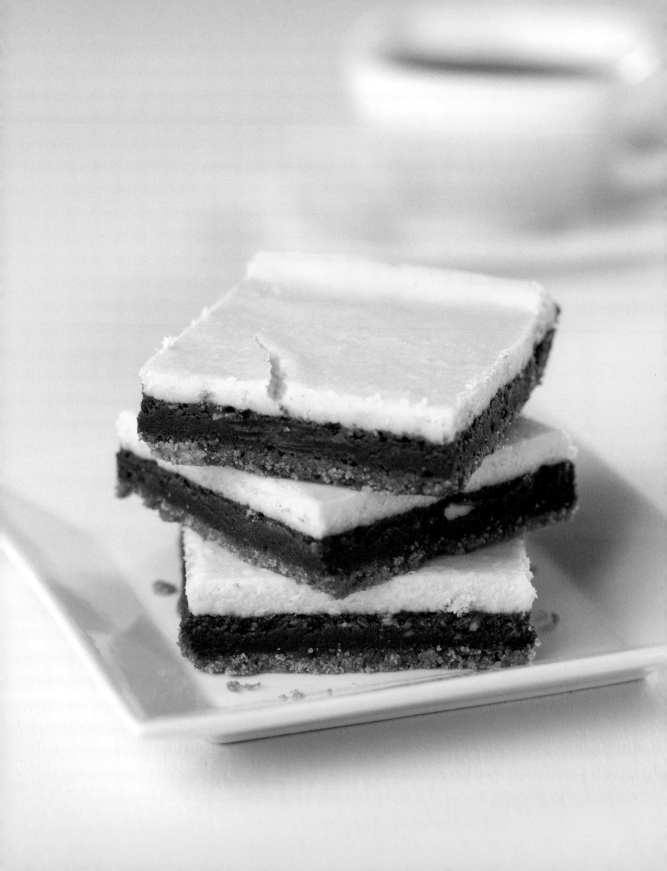

OMG! Brownie Cheesecake Bars

....

Want to meet your Higher Power? Then give some attention to this award-winning star. I pair a crunchy graham cracker crust and a deep, dark chocolate filling with a sublime layer of creamy cheesecake. The first time we made this at Sweet Mary Jane, one of our testers took a bite and blurted out, "OMG! Really?" Yes, really! This taste-of-heaven, melt-in-your-mouth, mind-blowing treat will bring you to the point of no return. And that's a good thing.

Makes 12 bars

THC per serving: Please see page 54 to calculate.

Vegetable shortening, for greasing the pan

Graham Cracker Crust

⅔ cup graham cracker crumbs (from about 8 or 9 graham crackers)

⅓ cup finely chopped walnuts, toasted

3 tablespoons sugar

¼ cup Buddha Budda (page 43), melted

Dark Chocolate Filling

6 ounces bittersweet chocolate

2 ounces cream cheese, slightly softened

3 tablespoons Buddha Budda (page 43), slightly softened

¾ cup sugar

2 large eggs

2 teaspoons pure vanilla extract

¼ teaspoon salt

½ cup sifted all-purpose flour

Cream Cheese Topping

9 ounces cream cheese, slightly softened

2 tablespoons Buddha Budda (page 43), slightly softened

1 tablespoon pure vanilla extract

½ cup sugar

2 large eggs

3 tablespoons whole milk

1 tablespoon all-purpose flour

1. Preheat the oven to 350°F. Grease a 9 x 13-inch baking pan with vegetable shortening and line it with foil, pressing it into the corners and letting about 3 inches hang over two opposite sides of the pan. Grease the foil.

2. Prepare the graham cracker crust: In the bowl of a food processor, combine the graham cracker crumbs, walnuts, and sugar and pulse until the walnuts are finely ground. Add the melted Buddha Budda and pulse to mix well. Press the mixture evenly over the bottom of the prepared baking pan. (Set the food processor bowl aside—you're going to use it again.) Bake for 6 to 8 minutes, until golden brown around the edges. Transfer to a wire rack to cool (leave the oven on).

3. Prepare the dark chocolate filling: In the top section of a double boiler, melt the chocolate over simmering water. Turn off the heat.

4. In a large bowl using an electric mixer, beat together the cream cheese and Buddha Budda until smooth. Mix in the sugar and combine well. Add the eggs one at a time, beating well after each addition. Stir in the vanilla, salt, and melted chocolate and combine well. Fold in the flour. Gently spread the filling evenly over the cooled crust.

5. Prepare the cream cheese topping: In the bowl of a food processor, combine the cream cheese, Buddha Budda, vanilla, and sugar and process until creamy. Add the eggs, milk, and flour and process until smooth. Carefully pour the cream cheese topping over the chocolate filling, tilting the pan to completely cover the chocolate with the topping.

6. Bake for 30 to 40 minutes, or until the top is dry but the center remains slightly soft and the edges begin to pull away from the sides of the pan.

Let cool completely on a wire rack. Cover and refrigerate for 8 hours or overnight.

7. Using the overhanging foil, lift out of the pan and place on a cutting board. Cut into 12 equal-size bars with a thin, sharp knife, dipping it in hot water before each cut. Wrap tightly in aluminum foil and store in the refrigerator for up to 5 days, or in the freezer for up to 3 months.

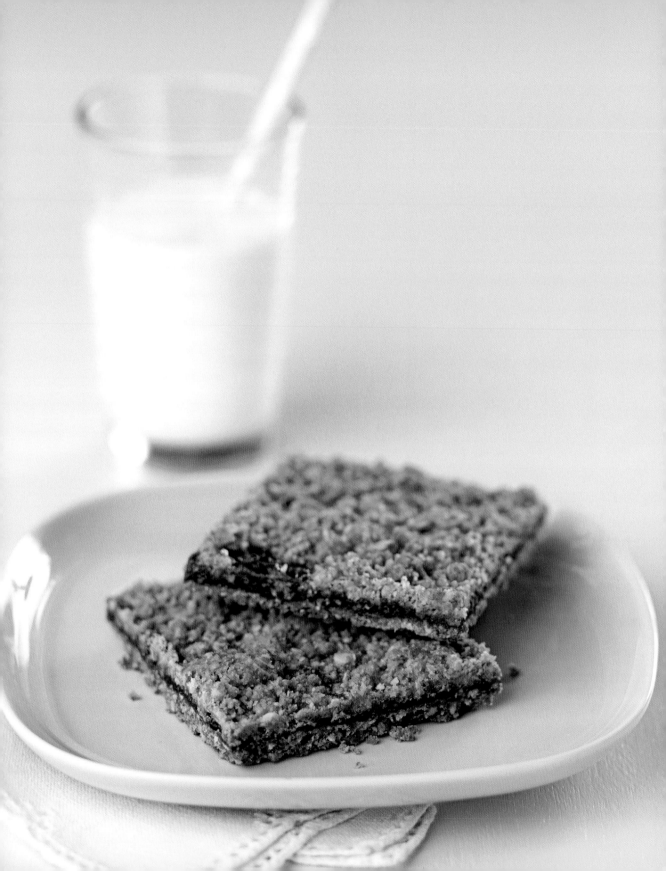

Raspberry Jam Session

Spread the love with a sweet and buttery raspberry jam breakfast bar with a short-bread crust and a streusel topping.

Makes 12 bars

THC per serving: Please see page 54 to calculate.

Vegetable shortening, for greasing the pan
1½ cups all-purpose flour
1 cup firmly packed dark brown sugar
1 cup old-fashioned rolled oats
¾ cup pecans
1 teaspoon salt
¾ teaspoon baking powder
½ teaspoon baking soda
2 teaspoons ground cinnamon
½ cup Buddha Budda (page 43)
¼ cup (4 tablespoons/½ stick) unsalted butter
1 cup raspberry jam (see Note, page 78)

1. Preheat the oven to 350°F. Grease a 9 x 13-inch baking pan and line it with foil, pressing it into the corners and letting about 3 inches hang over two opposite sides of the pan.

2. In the bowl of a food processor, combine the flour, brown sugar, oats, pecans, salt, baking powder, baking soda, and cinnamon, and pulse in short bursts until combined. Add the Buddha Budda and butter and pulse until well incorporated. Take out 1½ cups of the mixture and set it aside.

3. Transfer the rest of the mixture to the prepared pan and press it into an even layer. Bake for 12 to 15 minutes, until golden brown. Transfer to a wire rack to cool (leave the oven on).

4. Spread the raspberry jam over the cooled crust and top with the reserved crumb mixture, pressing it gently into the jam. Bake for 35 to 45 minutes, until the topping is golden brown and the filling starts to bubble around the edges. Transfer to a wire rack to cool completely.

5. Using the overhanging foil, gently lift out of the pan and place on a cutting board. Cut into 12 equal-size bars. Wrap tightly in aluminum foil and store in the refrigerator for up to 1 week, or in the freezer for up to 3 months.

Note: *Crofters Organic Just Fruit Spread works beautifully here; it's not too sweet, spreads easily, and is organic. But this is a forgiving bar and any jam or spread will work. It doesn't even have to be raspberry.*

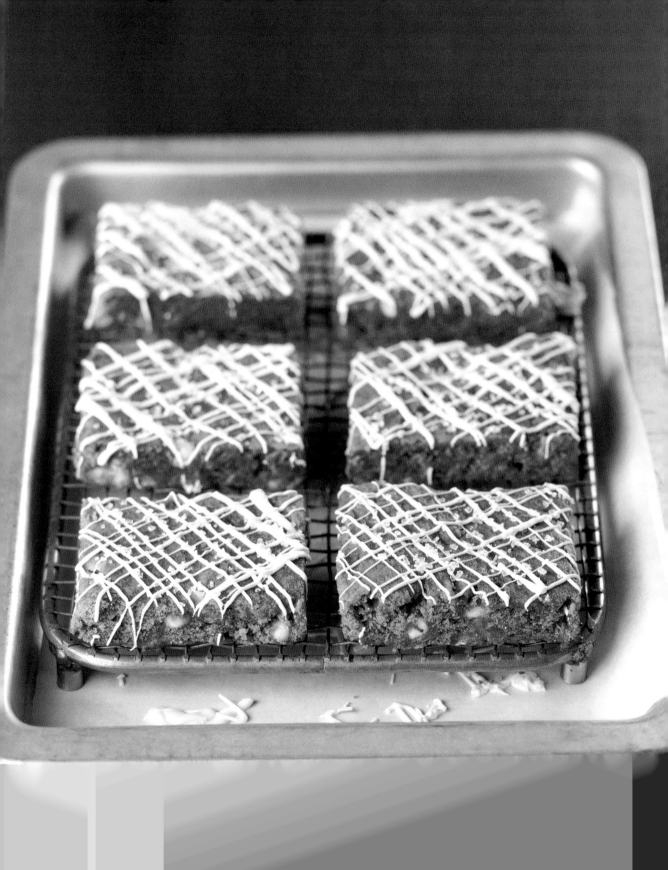

Smashing Pumpkin Bars

....

Originally, I thought Smashing Pumpkin Bars were going to be a seasonal treat. But then we started getting orders for them in January. And then April. And then July. I guess they're an anytime treat! Bonus: They make your kitchen smell like heaven.

Makes 18 bars

THC per serving: Please see page 54 to calculate.

Vegetable shortening, for greasing the pan
2 cups all-purpose flour
2 teaspoons ground cinnamon
½ teaspoon ground cloves
½ teaspoon ground allspice
½ teaspoon freshly grated nutmeg
½ teaspoon salt
½ cup Buddha Budda (page 43), slightly softened
½ cup (8 tablespoons/1 stick) unsalted butter, slightly softened
½ cup firmly packed dark brown sugar
½ cup granulated sugar
1 large egg
1 tablespoon pure vanilla extract
1 cup pure pumpkin puree
¾ cup white chocolate chips
½ cup pecans, coarsely chopped, toasted (optional)
⅓ cup dried cranberries (optional)

Glaze
6 ounces white chocolate chips
2 teaspoons vegetable shortening

Clear sugar sprinkles

1. Preheat the oven to 350°F. Grease a 10 x 15-inch baking pan with vegetable shortening.

2. In a medium bowl, whisk together the flour, cinnamon, cloves, allspice, nutmeg, and salt; set aside.

3. In a large bowl using an electric mixer, cream together the Buddha Budda, butter, brown sugar, and granulated sugar on medium speed until light and fluffy. Beat in the egg and vanilla. Add the pumpkin and combine well. Reduce the mixer speed to low and add the flour mixture. Beat well. Fold in the white chocolate chips and, if using, the pecans and cranberries. Pour the batter into the prepared pan and smooth it into an even layer using an offset spatula.

4. Bake until a toothpick inserted into the center comes out clean, 18 to 22 minutes. Transfer the pan to a wire rack to cool completely. Cut into 18 equal-size bars.

5. Prepare the glaze: In the top section of a double boiler, melt the white chocolate and shortening over simmering water. Stir continuously until the chocolate has melted, being careful not to get any water into the chocolate or it will seize (see Note).

6. Remove the brownies from the pan and place them on a wire rack set over waxed paper. Dip a fork into the glaze and drizzle it over the brownies in a crisscross pattern. Dust the brownies with clear sugar sprinkles.

7. Wrap tightly in aluminum foil and store in the refrigerator for up to 1 week, or in the freezer for up to 3 months.

Note: Chocolate should melt into a smooth, satiny pool, but it's temperamental and will not tolerate moisture. If even the tiniest bit of condensation drips down the inside of a pan, or if steam escapes from the bottom of the double boiler, the chocolate will react badly, becoming a grainy mess; this is known as "seizing."

Walnut Fantasy

Rich, dark, and brimming with walnuts—you'll score brownie points with this one. I was making these long before starting Sweet Mary Jane—I can't even remember where the original recipe came from. But little by little, it has changed. At first I used semisweet chocolate for the base, but with the caramelized topping the whole thing was overly sweet. So I switched to unsweetened chocolate, and it made a world of difference. I've tried this with a variety of nuts—toasted pecans, toasted almonds, even pine nuts (so amenable, this one)—but the walnut topping is by far my favorite.

This recipe is a great one for gluten-free baking (just substitute gluten-free flour; at Sweet Mary Jane, we use almond flour or rice flour) and is a constant on our De-Floured (say it out loud) menu. If you are lactose-intolerant, substitute Coconut Bliss for the Buddha Budda.

Makes 12 brownies

THC per serving: Please see page 54 to calculate.

Brownie Base

Vegetable shortening, for greasing
   the pan
6 tablespoons Buddha Budda (page 43)
3 ounces unsweetened chocolate
1 cup sugar

¼ teaspoon salt
2 large eggs, lightly beaten
2 teaspoons pure vanilla extract
½ cup all-purpose flour

Caramelized Walnut Topping

2 tablespoons Buddha Budda (page 43)
2 tablespoons unsalted butter
¼ cup granulated sugar
½ cup firmly packed light brown sugar

2 tablespoons all-purpose flour
2 large eggs, lightly beaten
1 tablespoon pure vanilla extract
3½ cups coarsely chopped walnuts

1. Prepare the brownie base: Grease a 9 x 9-inch baking pan with vegetable shortening and line it with foil, pressing it into the corners and letting about 3 inches hang over two opposite sides of the pan. Grease the foil.

2. In a medium saucepan, melt the Buddha Budda over low heat. Add the chocolate and stir continuously until melted. Remove from the heat. Stir in the sugar and salt. Add the eggs and vanilla and combine well. Fold in the flour. Pour the batter evenly into the prepared pan. Place in the refrigerator for 2 hours or overnight.

3. Preheat the oven to 350°F.

4. Prepare the topping: In a medium saucepan, melt the Buddha Budda and butter together over low heat. Stir in the granulated and brown sugars and cook, stirring continuously, for 1 minute. Remove from the heat. Add the flour and eggs and blend well. Return to the stovetop over low heat. Cook, stirring continuously to prevent the eggs from curdling, for 3 minutes. Remove from the heat and add the vanilla and walnuts. Spoon the topping over the chilled brownie base, spreading it evenly to the edges of the pan.

5. Bake for 40 to 50 minutes, until a toothpick inserted 2 inches from the center comes out with a few crumbs clinging to it and the topping is dry. Transfer to a wire rack to cool completely. Cover and refrigerate for 8 hours or overnight.

6. Using the overhanging foil, gently lift out of the pan and set on a cutting board. Cut into 12 equal-size bars. Wrap tightly in aluminum foil and store in the refrigerator for up to 1 week, or in the freezer for up to 3 months.

Mark T's Raw Bar Yogi Treats

Vegan, Raw

The raw food movement is big here in Boulder, but I noticed that there were no cannabis-infused raw products available. So I created these for my dear friend and yogi extraordinaire Mark. Cut them into 24 pieces and pop a bite-size snack into your mouth whenever you desire. Raw inspiring!

Makes 24 pieces

THC per serving: Please see page 54 to calculate.

Vegetable shortening, for greasing the pan
½ cup honey
¼ cup Coconut Bliss (page 46)
¼ cup almond butter
2 ounces unsweetened chocolate, grated
1 cup slivered almonds, coarsely chopped
½ cup mixed seeds, such as hemp, pepitas, chia, and sunflower
¼ cup dried cherries
2 tablespoons cacao nibs
1 cup old-fashioned rolled oats
¼ teaspoon sea salt

1. Grease an 8 x 8-inch baking pan with vegetable shortening.

2. In a medium saucepan, warm the honey, Coconut Bliss, and almond butter over low heat, no higher than 104°F. Add the chocolate and stir until the chocolate has melted and the mixture is smooth. Remove from the heat.

3. Stir in the remaining ingredients. Transfer the mixture to the prepared pan and press into an even layer. Cover and refrigerate for 2 hours.

4. Cut into 24 pieces. Wrap tightly in aluminum foil and store in the refrigerator for up to 1 month.

COOKIES

BETTER BUDDER PEANUT BUTTER COOKIES · *88*

BIG BHANG! COOKIES · *91*

CARROT CAKE COOKIES · *93*

CHOCOLATE SUPREMES · *97*

FEEL THE LOVE LEMON SANDWICH COOKIES · *99*

LUCIE IN THE SKY · *103*

HIGH-END CELESTIAL COOKIES · *107*

POP ROCKS SANDWICH COOKIES · *111*

BIG S OATMEAL COOKIES · *115*

FRENCH KISS TOASTED MACAROONS · *117*

ZO-ZO SNAPS · *119*

Better Budder Peanut Butter Cookies

Peanut butter and cannabis are an amazing combination, but if you toss in a little dark chocolate, it elevates this cookie to ohmygosh level. This grown-up version of peanut butter cookies is sexy and a bit mysterious. Sweet relief! Need I say more?

Makes 12 cookies

THC per serving: Please see page 54 to calculate.

Vegetable shortening, for greasing the baking sheets (optional)
1½ cups all-purpose flour
½ teaspoon baking powder
½ teaspoon baking soda
¾ teaspoon ground cinnamon
¼ teaspoon freshly grated nutmeg
¾ teaspoon coarse sea salt
½ cup Buddha Budda (page 43), slightly softened
½ cup creamy or chunky natural peanut butter
½ cup granulated sugar
½ cup firmly packed light brown sugar
1 large egg
2 teaspoons pure vanilla extract
¾ cup dark chocolate chips
Coarse sea salt, for sprinkling

1. Weigh the bowl that you will be using to hold the finished batter and write down this number. Preheat the oven to 375°F. Grease two baking sheets with vegetable shortening, or line them with parchment paper.

2. In a medium bowl, combine the flour, baking powder, baking soda, cinnamon, nutmeg, and salt. Set aside.

3. In a large bowl using an electric mixer, cream together the Buddha Budda, peanut butter, and granulated and brown sugars on medium speed until fluffy. Add the egg and vanilla and beat until smooth. Fold in the flour mix-

ture and combine well. Fold in the chips. Place the dough in the refrigerator for 1 hour.

4. Weigh the batter, subtract the weight of the bowl, and divide by 12: This is your per-cookie weight. Place a small piece of parchment paper on your scale. Weigh out the batter for each cookie and place the batter on the prepared baking sheet, spacing the cookies 4 inches apart. Flatten each cookie using the tines of a fork to create a crisscross pattern. Sprinkle each cookie with a bit of coarse sea salt.

5. Bake the cookies, one baking sheet at a time, until lightly golden around the edges, 8 to 10 minutes. Using a metal spatula, transfer the cookies to a wire rack and let cool.

6. Wrap tightly in aluminum foil and store in the refrigerator for up to 1 week, or in the freezer for up to 3 months.

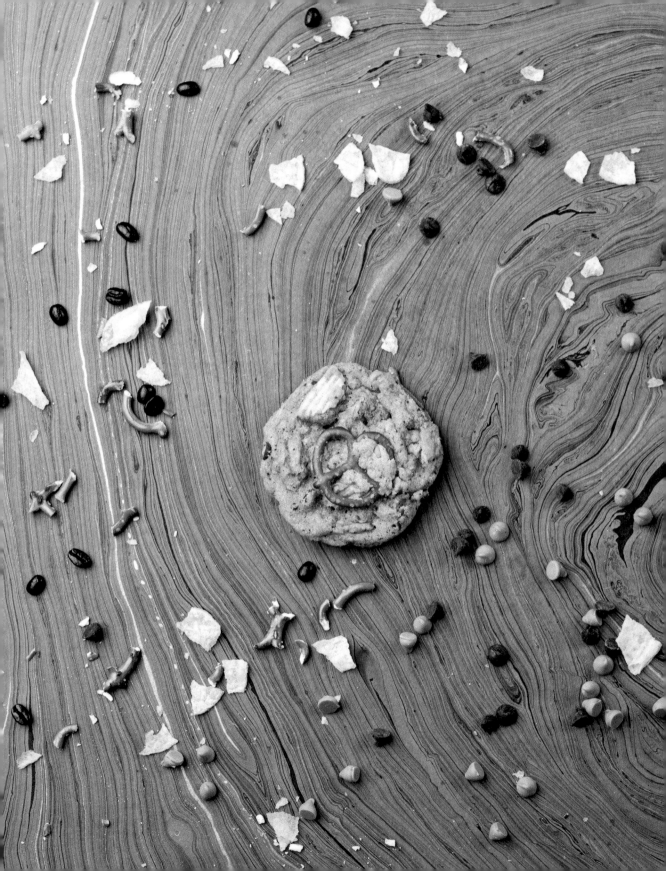

Big Bhang! Cookies

Potato chips, chocolate, butterscotch, pretzels! It's a volcanic taste explosion. (Thank you, Christina Tosi of Momofuku Milk Bar—you are a genius. I so adored your Compost Cookie, it became the inspiration for the Big Bhang!)

Makes 12 cookies

THC per serving: Please see page 54 to calculate.

Vegetable shortening, for greasing the baking sheets (optional)
½ cup Buddha Budda (page 43), slightly softened
½ cup granulated sugar
⅓ cup light brown sugar
1½ teaspoons corn syrup
1 small egg
½ teaspoon pure vanilla extract
¾ cup all-purpose flour
¼ teaspoon baking powder
⅛ teaspoon baking soda
½ teaspoon kosher or coarse sea salt
½ cup semisweet chocolate chips
¼ cup butterscotch chips
¼ cup graham cracker crumbs
¼ cup old-fashioned rolled oats
1¼ teaspoons freshly ground coffee beans
1 cup thick-cut potato chips, broken into ½- to 1-inch pieces
1 cup mini pretzels, coarsely chopped
½ cup Fritos

Drizzle
3 ounces semisweet chocolate
1 teaspoon vegetable shortening

1. Weigh the bowl that you will be using to hold the finished batter and write down this number. Grease two baking sheets with vegetable shortening, or line them with parchment paper.

2. In the bowl of a stand mixer fitted with the paddle attachment, cream together the Buddha Budda, granulated and brown sugars, and corn syrup on medium-high speed for 2 to 3 minutes. Scrape down the sides of the bowl, add the egg and vanilla, and beat for 7 to 8 minutes.

3. Reduce the mixer speed to low and add the flour, baking powder, baking soda, and salt. Mix just until the dough comes together. Add the chocolate chips, butterscotch chips, graham cracker crumbs, oats, and coffee and mix until just incorporated, about 30 seconds. Add the potato chips, pretzels, and Fritos and mix until just combined. Do not overmix.

4. Weigh the batter, subtract the weight of the bowl, and divide by 12: This is your per-cookie weight. Place a small piece of parchment paper on your scale. Weigh out the batter for each cookie and form each cookie into a disc. Place the cookies on the prepared baking sheets and with the palm of your hand, flatten each cookie to ¼ inch thick. Space the cookies at least 4 inches apart on the baking sheets. Wrap the baking sheets tightly with plastic wrap and refrigerate for 1 hour, or up to 1 week. (The cookies must be chilled before baking.)

5. When ready to bake, preheat the oven to 375°F. Bake the cookies, one sheet at a time, for 18 to 20 minutes, or until the cookies puff, crackle, and spread, and are golden brown on the edges. Let cool on the baking sheets before transferring to a wire rack to cool completely.

6. Prepare the drizzle: In the top section of a double boiler, melt the chocolate and shortening over simmering water. Stir well to combine. Drizzle a little over the top of each cookie. Let cool.

7. Wrap tightly in aluminum foil and store in the refrigerator for up to 1 week, or in the freezer for up to 3 months.

Carrot Cake Cookies

··

These seductive cookies could make a bunny's nose twitch—but there's no rabbit food here, only golden ribbons of carrots intertwined with tart cherries sandwiching a voluptuous cloud of creamy filling. Nibble away!

Makes 24 cookies or 12 sandwiches

THC per serving: Please see page 54 to calculate.

Vegetable shortening, for greasing the baking sheets (optional)

Cookies
2½ cups all-purpose flour
1 cup old-fashioned rolled oats
½ teaspoon baking soda
½ teaspoon baking powder
1 teaspoon ground cinnamon
½ teaspoon ground ginger
½ teaspoon freshly grated nutmeg
½ teaspoon salt
½ cup Buddha Budda (page 43)
½ cup granulated sugar
½ cup plus 2 tablespoons firmly packed light brown sugar
1 large egg
2 teaspoons pure vanilla extract
¾ cup grated peeled carrots (about 2½ carrots)
¾ cup dried cherries

Cream Cheese Filling
1½ tablespoons unsalted butter, slightly softened
6 ounces cream cheese, slightly softened
3 tablespoons vegetable shortening
¼ teaspoon pure vanilla extract
2½ cups powdered sugar

1. Prepare the cookies: Preheat the oven to 375°F. Weigh the bowl that you will be using to hold the finished batter and write down this number. Grease two baking sheets with vegetable shortening, or line them with parchment paper.

2. In a large bowl, combine the flour, oats, baking soda, baking powder, cinnamon, ginger, nutmeg, and salt. Set aside.

3. In a large bowl using an electric mixer, cream together the Buddha Budda and granulated and brown sugars on medium speed until light and fluffy. Add the egg and vanilla.

4. Reduce the mixer speed to low and add the flour mixture. Add the carrots and dried cherries and combine well.

5. Weigh the batter, subtract the weight of the bowl, and divide by 24: This is your per-cookie weight. Place a piece of parchment paper on your scale and weigh out the batter for each cookie. Place the batter on the prepared baking sheets, spacing the cookies 2 inches apart. Flatten them with the palm of your hand so that each cookie is about ¼ inch thick.

6. Bake the cookies, one sheet at a time, for 9 to 11 minutes, or until the tops are a light golden brown. Transfer to a wire rack to cool completely.

7. Prepare the cream cheese filling: In a large bowl using an electric mixer, cream the butter, cream cheese, shortening, and vanilla together on medium speed until smooth. Reduce the mixer speed to low and gradually add the powdered sugar, scraping down the sides of the bowl frequently. Beat until smooth.

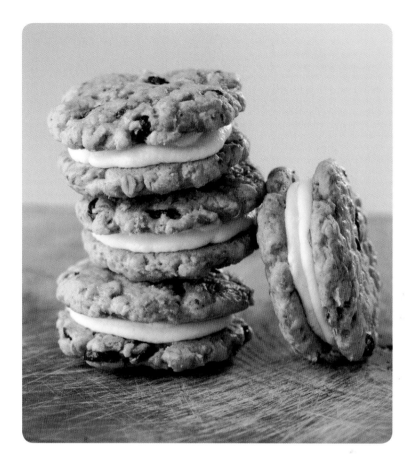

8. Pipe or spoon a dollop of the filling onto the flat side of half the cooled cookies and top with remaining cookies. If you are going to freeze these, don't fill the cookies. Defrost and then fill them.

9. Wrap tightly in aluminum foil and store in the refrigerator for up to 1 week, or in the freezer for up to 3 months.

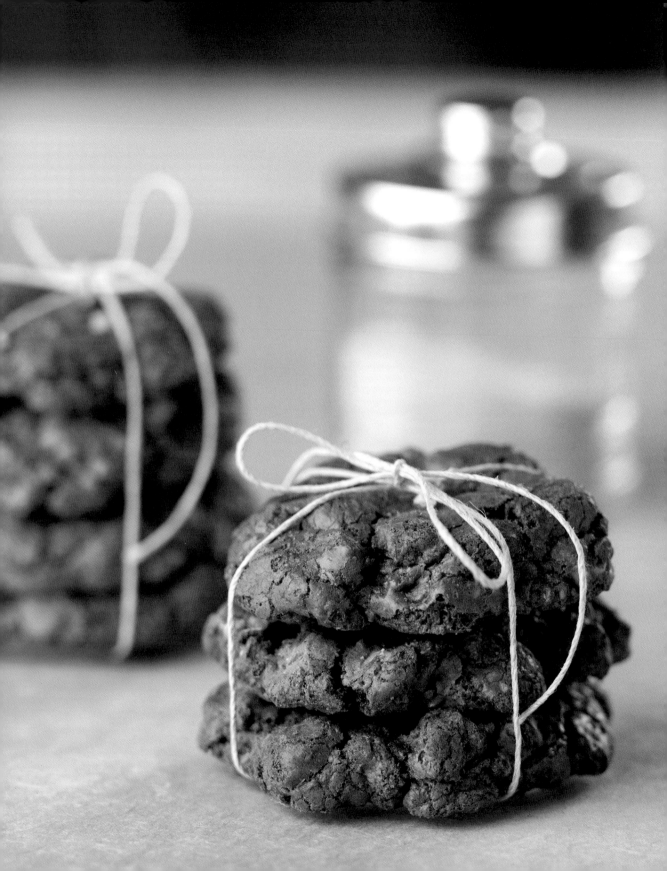

Chocolate Supremes

This delicious recipe yields a rich, molten mass somewhere between a gooey brownie and a luscious cookie.

Makes 18 cookies

THC per serving: Please see page 54 to calculate.

Vegetable shortening, for greasing the baking sheets (optional)
6 ounces bittersweet chocolate, finely chopped
2 ounces unsweetened chocolate, finely chopped
6 tablespoons (¾ stick) unsalted butter
1 tablespoon freshly ground espresso
½ cup all-purpose flour
1 teaspoon baking powder
¼ teaspoon salt
2 large eggs, at room temperature
6 tablespoons Hey Sugar! (page 51)
1 tablespoon granulated sugar
1 tablespoon pure vanilla extract
1 cup coarsely chopped pecans
1 cup coarsely chopped walnuts
6 ounces bittersweet chocolate, cut into ¼-inch chunks

1. Weigh the bowl that you will be using to hold the finished batter and write down this number. Grease two baking sheets with vegetable shortening, or line them with parchment paper.

2. In the top section of a double boiler, combine the finely chopped chocolates, butter, and espresso and melt over simmering water, stirring occasionally until smooth. Set aside to cool slightly.

3. In a medium bowl, whisk together the flour, baking powder, and salt. Set aside.

4. In the bowl of a stand mixer fitted with the paddle attachment, combine the eggs and Hey Sugar! and whip until the mixture is light in color and increases substantially in volume, about 10 minutes. Beat in the vanilla. Stir in the melted chocolate. Fold in the flour mixture until just combined. Stir in the pecans, walnuts, and chocolate chunks. Cover and refrigerate the dough for 1 hour.

5. Preheat the oven to 325°F.

6. Weigh the batter, subtract the weight of the bowl, and divide by 18: This is your per-cookie weight. Place a piece of parchment paper on your scale. Weigh out the batter for each cookie and drop the batter onto the prepared baking sheets, spacing 2 inches apart. Bake one sheet at a time until the cookies are slightly puffed and cracked on the outside but gooey inside, 8 to 11 minutes. Let cool on the baking sheets.

7. Wrap tightly in aluminum foil and store in the refrigerator for up to 1 week, or in the freezer for up to 3 months.

Feel the Love Lemon Sandwich Cookies

··

A tantalizingly tangy lemon filling sandwiched between two melt-in-your-mouth sugar cookies. Surprisingly easy to bake and even easier to eat!

Makes 6 sandwich cookies

THC per serving: Please see page 54 to calculate.

Tangy Lemon Curd Filling
¼ cup (4 tablespoons/½ stick) unsalted butter, slightly softened
¾ cup granulated sugar
1 tablespoon lemon zest
2 extra-large eggs
¼ cup fresh lemon juice (from 2 to 3 lemons)
⅛ teaspoon salt

Cookies
Vegetable shortening, for greasing the baking sheets (optional)
½ cup plus 2½ tablespoons all-purpose flour
⅓ cup cornstarch
¼ teaspoon salt
¼ cup Buddha Budda (page 43), slightly softened
¼ cup (4 tablespoons/½ stick) salted butter,
    slightly softened
¼ cup powdered sugar
2 teaspoons lemon zest
1 teaspoon pure vanilla extract
¼ cup raw sugar (you may add more to taste)

1. Prepare the tangy lemon curd filling: In a large bowl using an electric mixer, cream together the butter, sugar, and zest on medium speed. Add the eggs one at a time, then add the lemon juice and salt. Mix until combined.

2. Pour the mixture into a 1-quart saucepan and cook over low heat, stirring continuously, until thickened, about 10 minutes. The lemon curd will thicken at about 170°F, or just below a simmer. Remove from the heat and let cool to room temperature.

3. Prepare the cookies: Preheat the oven to 350°F. Weigh the bowl that you will be using to hold the finished batter and write down this number. Grease two baking sheets with vegetable shortening, or line them with parchment paper.

4. In a medium bowl, whisk together the flour, cornstarch, and salt. Set aside.

5. In a large bowl using an electric mixer, beat together the Buddha Budda, butter, and powdered sugar on medium speed until pale and fluffy. Beat in the lemon zest and vanilla. With the mixer on low speed, beat in the flour mixture just until a soft dough forms.

6. Put the raw sugar in a small shallow bowl. Weigh the batter, subtract the weight of the bowl, and divide by 12: This is your per-cookie weight. Place a piece of parchment paper on your scale. Weigh out the batter for each cookie, roll into a ball, and drop into the raw sugar, gently turning to coat. Transfer to the prepared baking sheets, spacing the cookies ¾ inch apart. Flatten slightly with the palm of your hand.

7. Bake the cookies, one sheet at a time, until the tops are slightly cracked but still pale, 12 to 15 minutes. Transfer the cookies to a wire rack to cool completely. Let cool completely before filling.

8. On the flat side of half the cookies, place 1 rounded teaspoon of the filling. Refrigerate the cookies until the curd is set, 15 to 20 minutes, then top with the remaining cookies. Refrigerate for 4 hours before serving. If you are going to freeze these, don't fill the cookies. Defrost and then fill them.

9. Wrap tightly in aluminum foil and store in the refrigerator for up to 1 week, or in the freezer for up to 3 months.

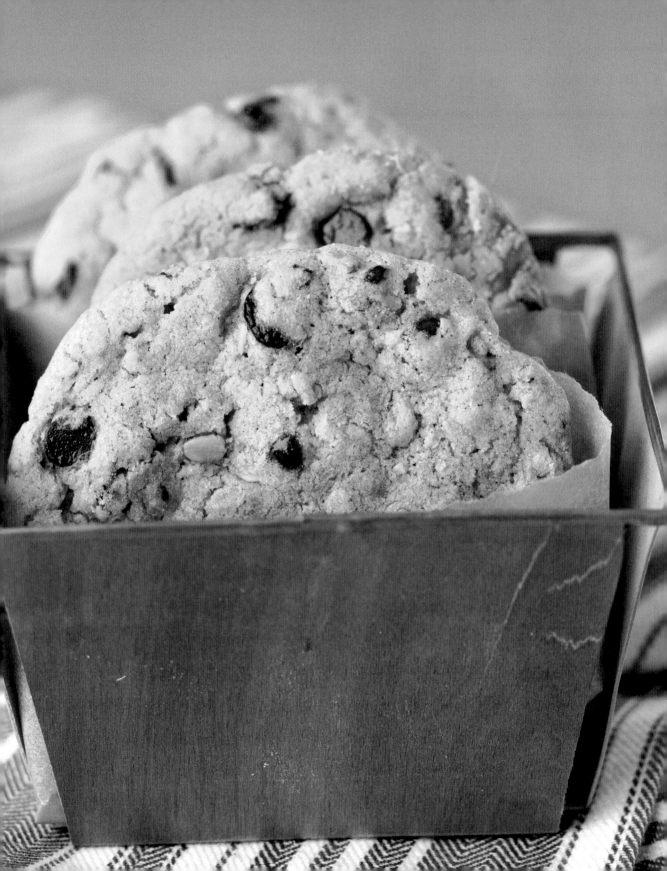

Lucie in the Sky

....

Chocolate chip cookies: Been there, ate that? Nope, not this one. Meet my daughter Lucie's version. She wasn't looking to reinvent the wheel—just, you know, change things up a bit. She added a whisper of cinnamon, some oats, and a handful of tart cranberries, bringing an everyday chocolate chip cookie from yum *all the way to* holy sh*t, that's delicious.

Makes 18 cookies

THC per serving: Please see page 54 to calculate.

Vegetable shortening, for greasing the baking sheets (optional)
1½ cups all-purpose flour
1 teaspoon baking soda
1 teaspoon ground cinnamon
½ teaspoon salt
1½ cups old-fashioned rolled oats
¾ cup Buddha Budda (page 43), slightly softened
¼ cup (4 tablespoons/½ stick) unsalted butter, slightly softened
¾ cup granulated sugar
¾ cup firmly packed light brown sugar
2 teaspoons pure vanilla extract
1 large egg
½ cup dried cranberries
½ cup bittersweet or semisweet chocolate chips

1. Weigh the bowl that you will be using to hold the finished batter and write down this number. Grease two baking sheets with vegetable shortening, or line them with parchment paper.

2. In a large bowl, stir together the flour, baking soda, cinnamon, salt, and oats. Set aside.

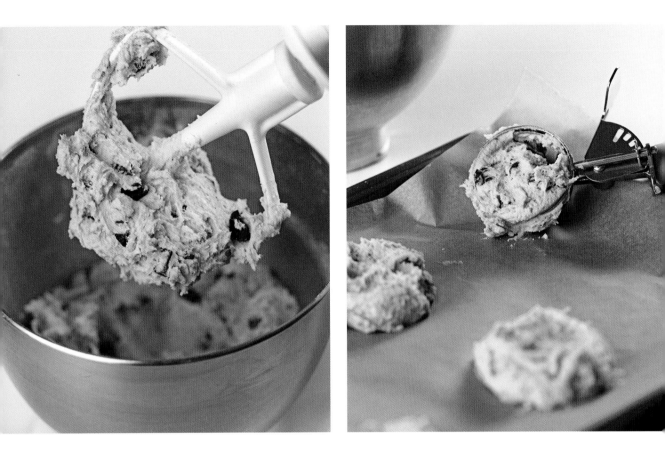

3. In a separate large bowl using an electric mixer, cream together the Buddha Budda, butter, and granulated and brown sugars on medium speed until light and fluffy. Add the vanilla and egg and beat until well combined. Add the flour mixture and beat until just combined. Fold in the cranberries and chocolate chips. Cover and refrigerate for 1 hour.

4. Preheat the oven to 375°F. Weigh the batter, subtract the weight of the bowl, and divide by 18: This is your per-cookie weight. Place a small piece of parchment paper on your scale. Weigh out the batter for each cookie and place the cookies on the prepared baking sheets, spacing them about

3 inches apart. Using the palm of your hand, flatten them to about ¼ inch thick.

5. Bake the cookies, one sheet at a time, for 10 to 12 minutes. They should be crispy on the outside and chewy on the inside.

6. Wrap tightly in aluminum foil and store in the refrigerator for up to 1 week, or in the freezer for up to 3 months.

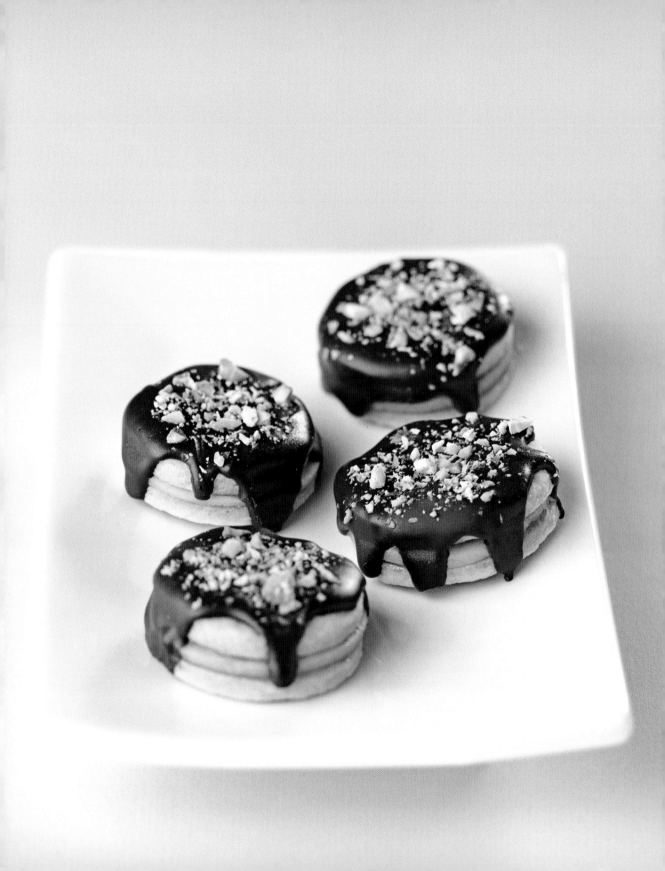

High-End Celestial Cookies

Look who's getting fancy. These cookies may seem complicated to prepare, but that's not really the case. Little wafers of sweetness are filled with apricot jam and almondy marzipan. Simple! And the taste? Out of this world!

Makes 24 sandwich cookies

THC per serving: Please see page 54 to calculate.

Vegetable shortening, for greasing the baking sheets (optional)

Cookies
½ cup Buddha Budda (page 43), slightly softened
1 cup granulated sugar
2 egg yolks
2 tablespoons fresh lemon juice
2½ cups all-purpose flour, plus more for dusting

Filling
5 tablespoons apricot jam
7 ounces marzipan
¾ cup powdered sugar

Glaze
6 ounces bittersweet chocolate, chopped
2 teaspoons vegetable shortening

4 ounces (½ cup) chopped salted pistachios, for garnish

1. Grease two baking sheets with vegetable shortening, or line them with parchment paper.

2. Prepare the cookies: In a large bowl using an electric mixer, cream together the Buddha Budda and sugar on medium speed until light and fluffy.

Add the egg yolks and lemon juice. Reduce the mixer speed to low, add the flour, and mix until combined. If the dough is dry, stir in 1 teaspoon water. Gather the dough into a ball, flatten it into a disc, wrap in plastic wrap, and chill for 1 hour.

3. Preheat the oven to 350°F.

4. Roll out the chilled dough on a floured surface until it is about 1/16 inch thick. Using a 2-inch-round cookie cutter, cut circles from the dough; reroll the trimmings until all the dough has been used. Place the cookies on the prepared baking sheets and refrigerate for 30 minutes.

5. Bake for 8 to 10 minutes or until lightly golden. Transfer to a wire rack to cool completely.

6. Meanwhile, prepare the filling: In a small saucepan, warm the apricot jam over medium heat until melted. Press the jam through a fine-mesh sieve into a bowl. Place a heaping ¼ teaspoon of the jam onto half of the cooled cookies, spreading the jam to the edges. If you are going to freeze these, don't fill or glaze the cookies. Defrost and then fill and glaze them.

7. In a medium bowl using an electric mixer, combine the marzipan with ¼ cup of the powdered sugar and beat on medium speed until well blended. Gather it into a ball and flatten. Dust a work surface with the remaining powdered sugar and roll out the marzipan mixture until it is about ⅛ inch thick. Cut out circles, using the same cookie cutter you used for the dough. Gently press the marzipan circles over the jam on the cookies. Place the remaining cookies on top and press them lightly together. Using a spatula, transfer the cookies to a wire rack set over a sheet of parchment paper.

8. Prepare the glaze: In the top section of a double boiler, melt the chocolate and shortening over simmering water until smooth. Pour the chocolate into a spouted measuring cup and pour a little over each cookie, covering the top and allowing some to drip down the sides. Sprinkle the pistachios evenly over all the cookies before the chocolate sets. Let set.

9. Wrap tightly in aluminum foil and store in the refrigerator for up to 1 week, or in the freezer for up to 3 months.

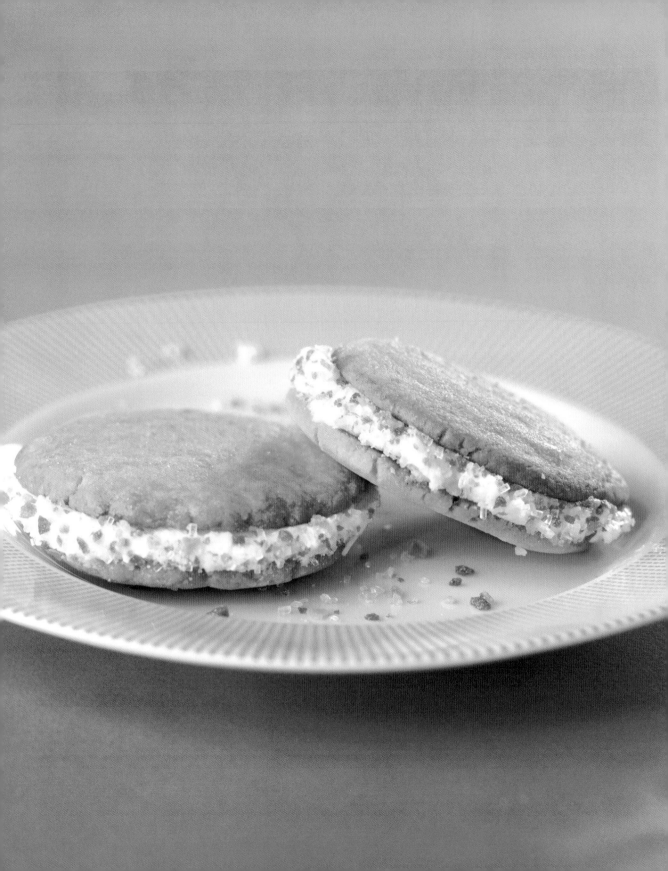

Pop Rocks Sandwich Cookies

Pop pop, fizz fizz, oh, what a relief it is—but the joy is in the surprise. Two cookies and a sparkly filling with a burst (really!) of flavor make this treat rock. At Sweet Mary Jane, we use chocolate- and cherry-flavored Pop Rocks, but feel free to go with your favorite flavor. To make this recipe gluten-free, substitute your favorite GF flour for the all-purpose flour, and make sure your powdered sugar is labeled gluten-free.

Makes 12 sandwich cookies

THC per serving: Please see page 54 to calculate.

Vegetable shortening, for greasing the baking sheets (optional)
2 cups all-purpose flour
¼ teaspoon freshly grated nutmeg
½ teaspoon baking soda
¼ teaspoon salt
½ cup Buddha Budda (page 43), slightly softened
¾ cup granulated sugar
¼ cup buttermilk
1 tablespoon pure vanilla extract

Cream Cheese Frosting
8 ounces cream cheese, slightly softened
½ cup (8 tablespoons/1 stick) salted butter, slightly softened
2 cups powdered sugar
2 teaspoons pure vanilla extract

2 (.33-ounce) bags Pop Rocks
Sparkly white or clear sprinkles (about ¼ cup, but you can always add more)

1. Weigh the bowl that you will be using to hold the finished batter and write down this number. Grease two baking sheets with vegetable shortening, or line them with parchment paper.

2. In a medium bowl, stir together the flour, nutmeg, baking soda, and salt.

3. In a large bowl using an electric mixer, cream together the Buddha Budda and sugar on medium speed until light and fluffy. Add the buttermilk and vanilla and beat until combined. The mixture may separate; don't worry, it will come together once the dry ingredients are added. Add the flour mixture and beat on low speed until combined. Cover and refrigerate for 30 minutes.

4. Preheat the oven to 350°F. Weigh the batter, subtract the weight of the bowl, and divide by 24: This is your per-cookie weight. Place a small piece of parchment paper on your scale. Weigh out the batter for each cookie and place the portions on the prepared baking sheet, spacing each cookie 2 inches apart. Gently flatten with the palm of your hand to about ⅛ inch thick.

5. Bake the cookies, one sheet at a time, for 8 to 10 minutes, or until lightly browned. Remove from the oven and let cool on the baking sheet on a wire rack. If you are going to freeze these, don't fill or coat the cookies. Defrost, fill, and then dip into the Pop Rocks mixture.

6. Prepare the frosting: In a large bowl using an electric mixer, beat the cream cheese and butter on medium-high speed until well combined. Reduce the mixer speed to low and gradually add the powdered sugar. When the mixture is fully incorporated, add the vanilla extract.

7. In a shallow bowl, combine the Pop Rocks and sprinkles. Once the cookies are cool, pipe or spoon a dollop of the frosting onto one cookie and top

with another. Dip the sides of each cookie sandwich in the Pop Rocks mixture and coat all the edges well.

8. Wrap tightly in aluminum foil and store in the refrigerator for up to 1 week, or in the freezer for up to 3 months.

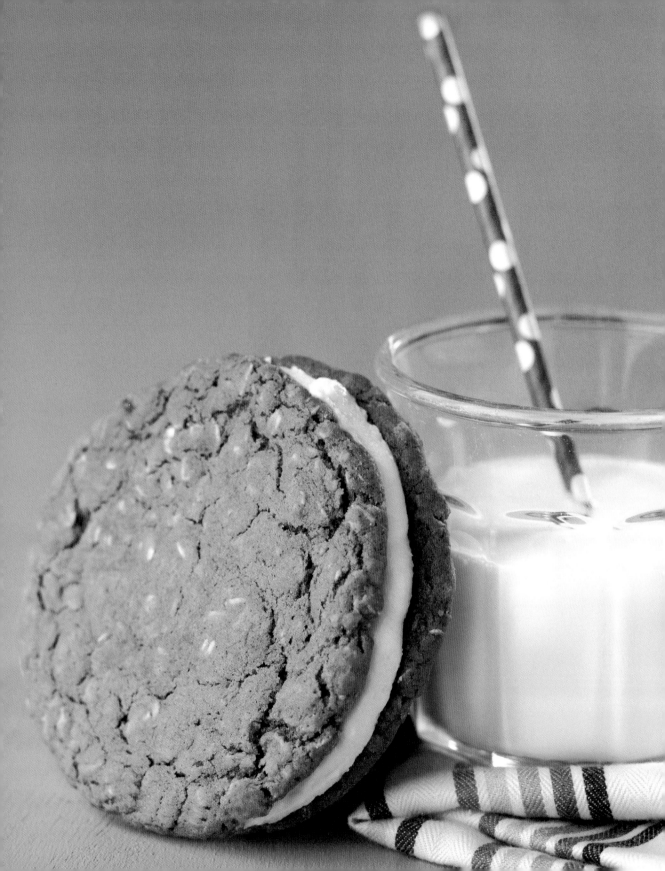

Big S Oatmeal Cookies

Remember the joy of after-school treats? Of course you do! This cookie has a sweetness that brings to mind the best childhood memories. And the name? Big S stands for Big Sandwich (of course!).

Makes 12 sandwich cookies

THC per serving: Please see page 54 to calculate.

Vegetable shortening, for greasing the baking sheets (optional)
2 cups firmly packed light brown sugar
1¼ teaspoons salt
2½ teaspoons ground cinnamon
½ cup (8 tablespoons/1 stick) unsalted butter, slightly softened
½ cup Buddha Budda (page 43), slightly softened
2 large eggs
¾ teaspoon baking soda
3 tablespoons unsulfured molasses
1½ teaspoons pure vanilla extract
3 cups old-fashioned rolled oats
3 cups all-purpose flour

Creamy Filling
3¾ cups sifted powdered sugar
1 cup vegetable shortening
Pinch of salt
¼ cup hot water
1½ teaspoons pure vanilla extract

1. Position a rack in the center of the oven and preheat to 350°F. Grease two baking sheets with vegetable shortening, or line them with parchment paper. Weigh the bowl that you will be using to hold the finished batter and write down this number.

2. In a bowl of a stand mixer fitted with the paddle attachment, beat together the brown sugar, salt, cinnamon, butter, and Buddha Budda on medium speed until light and fluffy, about 5 minutes. Beat in the eggs. In a small bowl, stir together the water and the baking soda until completely dissolved and add to the butter mixture. Blend in the molasses and scrape down the sides of the bowl as necessary. Add the vanilla. Add the oats, 1 cup at a time, scraping down the sides of the bowl as necessary, and blend thoroughly. Add the flour, 1 cup at a time, scraping down the sides of the bowl as necessary, and mix until incorporated.

3. Weigh the batter, subtract the weight of the bowl, and divide by 24: This is your per-cookie weight. Place a small piece of parchment paper on your scale. Weigh out the batter for each cookie and drop the batter onto the prepared baking sheets, spacing it 2 inches apart. Flatten the cookie dough with a spatula before baking. Bake the cookies, one sheet at a time, for 8 to 10 minutes, until light brown. Let cool completely before filling. If you are going to freeze these, don't fill the cookies. Defrost and then fill them.

4. Prepare the filling: In the bowl of a stand mixer fitted with the paddle attachment, combine the powdered sugar, shortening, and salt and mix on low speed until blended. Slowly add the hot water, then add the vanilla. Beat on medium-high speed until light and fluffy, about 5 minutes.

5. Pipe or spoon a dollop of the filling onto the flat side of half the cooled cookies. Top with the remaining cookies.

6. Wrap tightly in aluminum foil and store in the refrigerator for up to 1 week, or in the freezer for up to 3 months.

French Kiss Toasted Macaroons

Macaroons! Hey Sugar!, toasted coconut, and vanilla and almond extracts come to-gether in sweet harmony in this light-as-a-cloud treat. Considered a stroke of genius by the gluten-free crowd, those who do eat wheat also revel in them. I like to serve them with Mind Eraser Parfaits (page 202).

Makes 24 macaroons

THC per serving: Please see page 54 to calculate.

Vegetable shortening, for greasing the baking sheets (optional)
1 (14-ounce) package sweetened shredded coconut
3 large egg whites, at room temperature
¼ cup granulated sugar
¼ cup Hey Sugar! (page 51)
1 teaspoon pure vanilla extract
¼ teaspoon almond extract

1. Preheat the oven to 350°F. Grease a rimmed baking sheet with vegetable shortening, or line it with parchment paper. Place the coconut on the baking sheet and spread it evenly. Toast for 5 to 8 minutes, stirring every so often to ensure even color, until light golden brown. Let cool for 2 to 3 minutes.

2. Weigh the bowl that you will be using to hold the finished batter and write down this number. Grease two baking sheets with vegetable shorten-ing, or line them with parchment paper.

3. In a medium bowl using an electric mixer, beat the egg whites, granulated sugar, Hey Sugar!, and vanilla and almond extracts on high speed until the mixture becomes glossy, thick, and holds soft peaks. Fold in the toasted coconut.

4. Weigh the batter, subtract the weight of the bowl, and divide by 24: This is your per-cookie weight. Place a small piece of parchment paper on your scale. Using a small ice cream scoop, weigh out the batter for each cookie and place on the prepared baking sheet, spacing them 1 inch apart. Bake for 15 to 20 minutes, rotating the sheets halfway through, until golden brown. Let cool for 5 minutes on the baking sheet. Transfer to a wire rack and let cool completely.

5. The macaroons will keep in an airtight container at room temperature for up to 5 days, or you can freeze them for up to 3 months.

Zo-Zo Snaps

Zoe was the very first baker hired on at Sweet Mary Jane, and this is her cookie. It's sassy and might make you do bad things, like want to eat the whole batch. But don't. Seriously, don't.

Makes 15 cookies

THC per serving: Please see page 54 to calculate.

Vegetable shortening, for greasing the baking sheets (optional)
½ cup plus 2 tablespoons Buddha Budda (page 43), slightly softened
2 tablespoons unsalted butter, slightly softened
1 cup firmly packed dark brown sugar
1 large egg
¼ cup unsulfured molasses
1 tablespoon fresh or jarred minced ginger
2¼ cups all-purpose flour
2 teaspoons baking soda
½ teaspoon ground cinnamon
2 teaspoons ground ginger
¼ teaspoon ground cloves
¼ teaspoon salt
4 ounces bittersweet chocolate, shaved
⅓ to ½ cup raw sugar, plus more as necessary

1. Weigh the bowl that you will be using to hold the finished batter and write down this number. Grease two baking sheets with vegetable shortening, or line them with parchment paper.

2. In a large bowl using an electric mixer, cream together the Buddha Budda, butter, brown sugar, egg, molasses, and ginger on medium speed until light and fluffy. In a medium bowl, combine the flour, baking soda, cinnamon, ginger, cloves, and salt. Turn the mixer to low and fold in the flour mixture. Fold in the chocolate. Cover and refrigerate for 1 hour.

3. Preheat the oven to 375°F.

4. Weigh the batter, subtract the weight of the bowl, and divide by 15: This is your per-cookie weight. Place a small piece of parchment paper on your scale. Weigh out the batter for each cookie. Roll each cookie in the raw sugar and flatten with the palm of your hand to about ¼ inch thick. Place the cookies 4 inches apart on the baking sheets. Bake the cookies, one pan at a time, for 9 to 12 minutes, or until the tops are covered with little cracks. Let cool on a wire rack.

5. Wrap tightly in aluminum foil and store in the refrigerator for up to 1 week, or in the freezer for up to 3 months.

CAKES AND SWEET BREADS

ROSE PETAL SWEET BREAD • *122*

BLOOD ORANGE-GINGER SWEET BREAD • *125*

BERRY ENTERTAINING BLUEBERRY COFFEE CAKE • *127*

MAD BATTER CHOCOLATE CHIP COFFEE CAKE • *129*

CHOCOLATE THUNDER • *131*

JUST PEACHY COFFEE CAKE • *135*

MAPLE-PUMPKIN MOON PIES • *139*

Rose Petal Sweet Bread

··

Rose Petal Sweet Bread was one of my first "commercial" desserts. I came up with the recipe when I was in high school, one summer when the roses were in full bloom and their heady scent filled our backyard. I cut a few to bring into the kitchen and on a whim decided to sprinkle petals into a cake I was making. Lovely! Back then, I made and sold this treat without THC. You can infuse it by substituting Buddha Budda for regular butter. Or you can substitute ¼ cup Hey Sugar! for regular sugar.

Makes 12 servings

THC per serving: Please see page 54 to calculate.

½ cup (8 tablespoons/1 stick) unsalted butter, slightly softened,
     plus more for the pan
2½ cups all-purpose flour, plus more for the pan
2 teaspoons baking powder
1 cup sugar
2 large eggs
Zest of 1 orange
1 teaspoon pure vanilla extract
½ teaspoon rosewater
1 cup whole milk
½ cup pistachio nuts, coarsely chopped
½ cup unsprayed fresh rose petals, rinsed and dried

1. Preheat the oven to 350°F. Butter and flour an 8 x 4-inch loaf pan.

2. In a small bowl, stir together the flour and baking powder. Set aside.

3. In a large bowl using an electric mixer, cream together the butter and sugar on medium speed until light and fluffy. Add the eggs, orange zest, vanilla, and rosewater and beat until combined.

4. Reduce the mixer speed to low and add the flour mixture alternately with the milk, beginning and ending with the flour. Fold in the nuts and rose petals.

5. Bake for 40 to 45 minutes, until a toothpick inserted into the center of the bread comes out clean. Let cool in the pan for 10 minutes. Turn out onto a wire rack to cool completely. Cut into 12 equal-size slices.

6. Wrap tightly in aluminum foil and store in the refrigerator for up to 5 days, or in the freezer for up to 3 months.

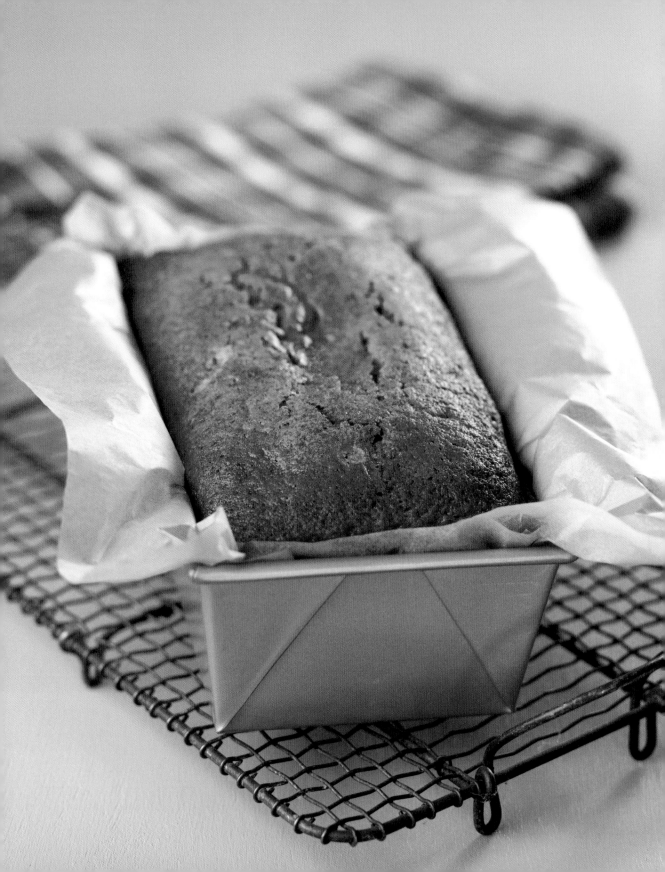

Blood Orange-Ginger Sweet Bread

Crimson-colored blood orange gives this cake its tangy twist. Spicy, nutty, and citrusy, with a crusty exterior and moist crumb, it makes for a perfect Sunday-morning brunch treat. Try it lightly toasted in the oven and slathered with butter.

Makes 8 big slices

THC per serving: Please see page 54 to calculate.

Vegetable shortening, for greasing the loaf pan
2 cups all-purpose flour
1 tablespoon Hey Sugar! (page 51)
1 cup granulated sugar
1½ teaspoons baking powder
½ teaspoon baking soda
½ teaspoon ground ginger
1 teaspoon ground cinnamon
1 teaspoon salt
¼ cup Buddha Budda (page 43), chilled
¾ cup apple cider
1 teaspoon almond extract
1 tablespoon blood orange zest
1 large egg
¼ cup coarsely chopped candied ginger
¾ cup peeled blood orange, chopped into ¼-inch pieces
½ cup slivered almonds, coarsely chopped
Powdered sugar, for dusting

1. Preheat the oven to 350°F. Grease the bottom and sides of a 9 x 5-inch loaf pan with vegetable shortening.

2. In a large bowl, stir together the flour, Hey Sugar!, granulated sugar, baking powder, baking soda, ground ginger, cinnamon, and salt. Cut the Buddha Budda into bits, then use your fingers to cut or rub it into the mixture until there are no pieces larger than a small pea.

3. In a medium bowl, whisk together the cider, almond extract, orange zest, and egg. Pour the cider mixture into the flour mixture, stirring just until the batter is moistened and smooth (do not overmix). Fold in the candied ginger, blood orange, and almonds; scrape the batter into the prepared loaf pan.

4. Bake for 55 to 65 minutes, or until the bread is golden brown and a toothpick inserted into the center comes out clean. Let cool on a wire rack for 15 minutes before removing from the pan. Dust with powdered sugar. Let cool completely before cutting into 8 equal-size slices.

5. Wrap tightly in aluminum foil and store in the refrigerator for up to 5 days, or in the freezer for up to 3 months.

Berry Entertaining Blueberry Coffee Cake

Bursting with lemon, cinnamon, and blueberry, this cake elicits visions of summer. But don't worry—you can make it in the depths of winter, too.

Makes 12 servings

THC per serving: Please see page 54 to calculate.

½ cup (8 tablespoons/1 stick) unsalted butter, slightly softened,
    plus more for the pan
3 cups all-purpose flour, plus more for the pan
1 tablespoon baking powder
1 teaspoon ground cinnamon
½ teaspoon salt
½ cup Buddha Budda (page 43), slightly softened
1½ cups granulated sugar
4 large eggs, at room temperature, lightly beaten
1 cup sour cream
2½ tablespoons lemon zest (from 4 large lemons)
2½ tablespoons fresh lemon juice (from 2 lemons)
1 tablespoon pure vanilla extract
¾ cup blueberry preserves
Powdered sugar, for dusting

1. Preheat the oven to 350°F. Butter and flour a 10-inch (14-cup) Bundt pan.

2. In a medium bowl, whisk together the flour, baking powder, cinnamon, and salt. Set aside.

3. In a large bowl using an electric mixer, beat together the butter and Buddha Budda on medium speed until creamy. Add the sugar and beat until light and fluffy. Beat in the eggs, sour cream, lemon zest, lemon juice, and vanilla. Reduce the mixer speed to low and add the flour mixture, beating until just incorporated.

4. Spread all but ½ cup of the batter into the prepared pan. Using the back of a spoon, make a well in the batter all the way around the pan. Mix the blueberry preserves with the reserved batter and spoon it into the well.

5. Bake for 1 to 1¼ hours, or until the cake begins to pull away from the pan and a skewer inserted into the center comes out clean. Let the cake cool in the pan for 15 minutes. Run a knife around the edge of the pan and invert the cake onto a wire rack. Sprinkle a light dusting of powdered sugar over the top. Slice into 12 equal-size pieces.

6. Wrap tightly in aluminum foil and store in the refrigerator for up to 1 week, or in the freezer for up to 3 months.

Mad Butter Chocolate Chip Coffee Cake

....

This easy-to-bake cake is the kind of thing you can make while lounging in your pj's on a weekend morning and enjoy later at brunch with friends. It's delicious warm from the oven, and perfect cold with a cup of tea or a glass of milk before bed.

Makes 12 servings

THC per serving: Please see page 54 to calculate.

½ cup (8 tablespoons/1 stick) unsalted butter, slightly softened,
    plus more for the pan
2¾ cups all-purpose flour, plus more for the pan
1 teaspoon salt
1 cup whole milk
2 teaspoons white vinegar
½ cup Buddha Budda (page 43), slightly softened
1 cup firmly packed dark brown sugar
1 tablespoon pure vanilla extract
4 large eggs
2 cups semisweet mini chocolate chips
¼ cup powdered sugar, for dusting

1. Preheat the oven to 375°F. Butter and flour a 10-inch Bundt pan.

2. In a small bowl, stir together the flour and salt. Set aside. In a separate small bowl, stir together the milk and vinegar. Set aside.

3. In a large bowl using an electric mixer, beat together the butter, Buddha Budda, brown sugar, and vanilla on medium speed until light and fluffy. Add the eggs one at a time, beating well after each addition. Reduce the mixer speed to low and gradually add the flour mixture, one-third at a time, alternating with the milk mixture. Gently fold in the chocolate chips. Pour into the prepared pan.

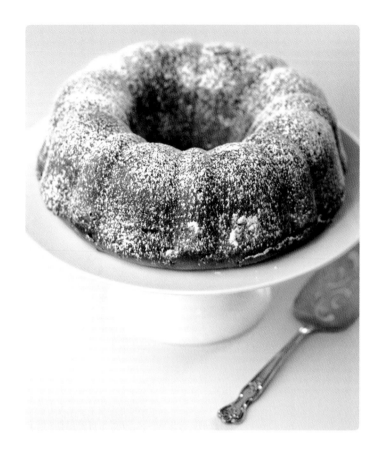

4. Bake for 40 to 50 minutes, or until a toothpick inserted into the center of the cake comes out clean. Let the pan cool on a wire rack for 20 minutes. Loosen the edges of the cake with a knife and invert onto a wire rack. Let cool completely. Pour the powdered sugar into a strainer and generously dust the top of the cake. Cut into 12 equal-size slices.

5. Wrap tightly in aluminum foil and store in the refrigerator for up to 1 week, or in the freezer for up to 3 months. You can freeze this either whole or in individual slices.

Chocolate Thunder

This cake is a crowd-pleaser, offering a subtle, grown-up balance of coffee, chocolate, and pistachios. I take a fabulously rich, layered, espresso-laced cake and cover it in a creamy, surprisingly deep- and complex-tasting chocolate frosting.

Makes 12 servings

THC per serving: Please see page 54 to calculate.

Vegetable shortening, for greasing the baking pan
2 tablespoons sifted unsweetened cocoa powder

Cake
½ cup Buddha Budda (page 43)
¼ cup (4 tablespoons/½ stick) unsalted butter
6 ounces bittersweet chocolate
1 teaspoon espresso powder
⅜ cup all-purpose flour
1 teaspoon salt
¾ cup sugar
4 large eggs
1 tablespoon pure vanilla extract

Ganache
8 ounces semisweet chocolate chips
1 cup heavy cream
2 tablespoons brewed espresso

1 cup salted pistachio nuts, coarsely chopped

1. Prepare the cake: Preheat the oven to 350°F. Line an 8 x 8-inch pan with aluminum foil, pressing it smoothly into all corners and leaving 3 inches hanging over two opposite sides. Grease the foil with vegetable shortening, and dust the bottom and sides with the cocoa powder, tapping out the excess.

2. In a small saucepan, melt the Buddha Budda, butter, and bittersweet chocolate over medium-low heat, stirring often until smooth, 4 to 5 minutes. Stir in the espresso powder. Set aside to cool to room temperature.

3. In a medium bowl, whisk together the flour and salt. Set aside.

4. In a large bowl using an electric mixer, beat together the sugar and eggs on medium speed until thick and pale yellow, 3 to 4 minutes. Add the vanilla and beat again until combined. Reduce the mixer speed to low and gradually add the flour mixture, beating until just combined. Add the melted chocolate mixture in a steady stream, beating until thoroughly blended. Transfer the batter to the prepared pan and smooth out the top.

5. Bake until a toothpick inserted near the edge of the cake comes out clean, about 25 minutes. Set aside to cool completely.

6. Meanwhile, prepare the ganache: Place the semisweet chocolate in a large, heat-proof bowl. In a small saucepan, heat the heavy cream until simmering. Pour the cream over the chocolate and stir gently until the chocolate has melted and the mixture is smooth. Stir in the espresso. Set aside and let cool to room temperature.

7. Lift the cake from the pan using the foil handles. Invert the cake onto a cutting board; peel off and discard the foil. Cut the cake in half horizontally to make two equal-size pieces. Invert one piece onto a wire rack set over a baking sheet. Spread with a generous layer of the ganache and sprinkle with half the pistachios. Top with the second cake layer, inverted so that it sits right-side up. Use the remaining ganache to cover the top and sides and

sprinkle with the remaining pistachios. Refrigerate, uncovered, until set, at least 2 hours and up to 2 days.

8. Cut into 12 equal-size slices. Wrap tightly in aluminum foil and store in the refrigerator for up to 5 days, or in the freezer for up to 3 months.

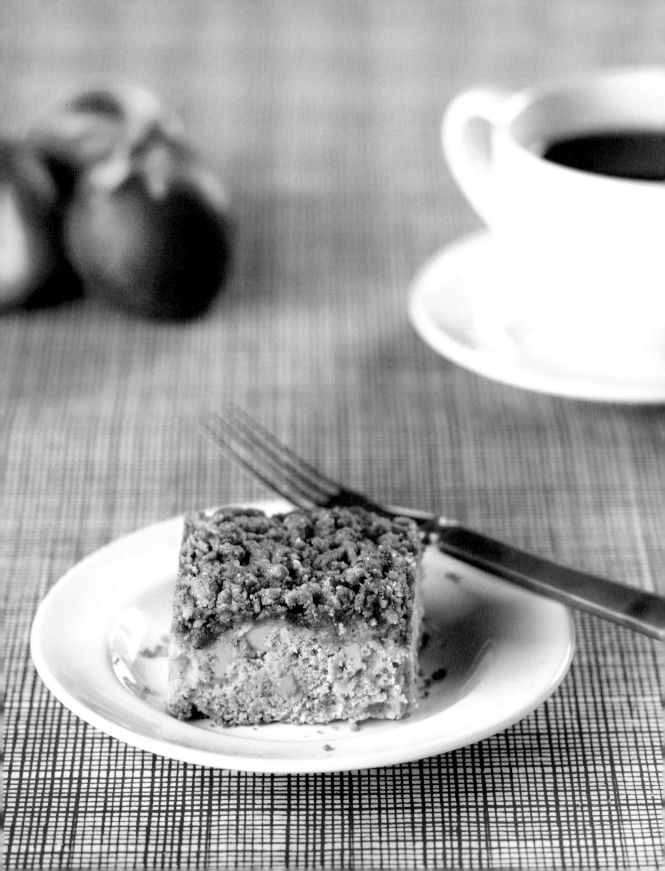

Just Peachy Coffee Cake

Make this cake first thing in the morning, and your house will smell like heaven on earth. Serve it right out of the oven. Sweet awakenings!

Makes 12 servings

THC per serving: Please see page 54 to calculate.

Vegetable shortening, for greasing the baking pan

Cake
2 cups all-purpose flour
2 teaspoons baking powder
½ teaspoon salt
2 teaspoons ground cinnamon
½ cup Buddha Budda (page 43), slightly softened
½ cup granulated sugar
2 large eggs
½ cup whole milk
1 teaspoon pure vanilla extract
1½ cups diced peaches (fresh or frozen)

Topping
½ cup (8 tablespoons/1 stick) unsalted butter
1 cup packed light brown sugar
¾ cup all-purpose flour
½ teaspoon salt
1 teaspoon freshly grated nutmeg
1 tablespoon ground cinnamon
1 cup pecans, chopped

1. Preheat the oven to 375°F. Grease a 9 x 13-inch cake pan.

2. Prepare the cake: In a large bowl, whisk together the flour, baking powder, salt, and cinnamon. Set aside.

3. In a separate large bowl using an electric mixer, beat together the Buddha Budda and granulated sugar on medium speed until light and fluffy. Add the eggs, milk, and vanilla. Slowly add the flour mixture and beat until smooth. Using a rubber spatula, gently fold in the peaches. Pour the batter into the prepared pan and smooth the top using a rubber spatula.

4. Prepare the topping: In a separate bowl, combine the butter, brown sugar, flour, salt, nutmeg, cinnamon, and pecans with a pastry cutter or your hands until crumbly. Sprinkle the topping evenly over the batter.

5. Bake for 25 to 35 minutes, or until a toothpick inserted into the center of the cake comes out clean. Let cool on a wire rack for 15 minutes. Cut into 12 equal-size pieces.

6. Wrap tightly in aluminum foil and store in the refrigerator for up to 5 days, or in the freezer for up to 3 months.

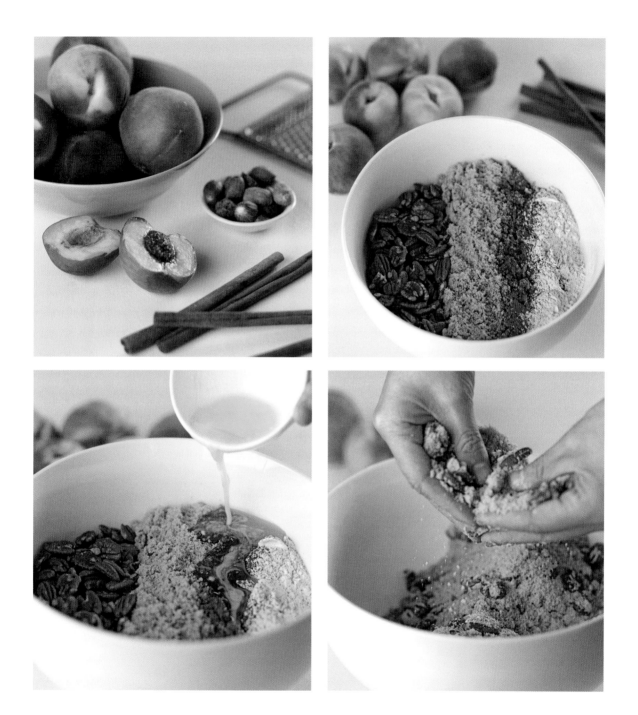

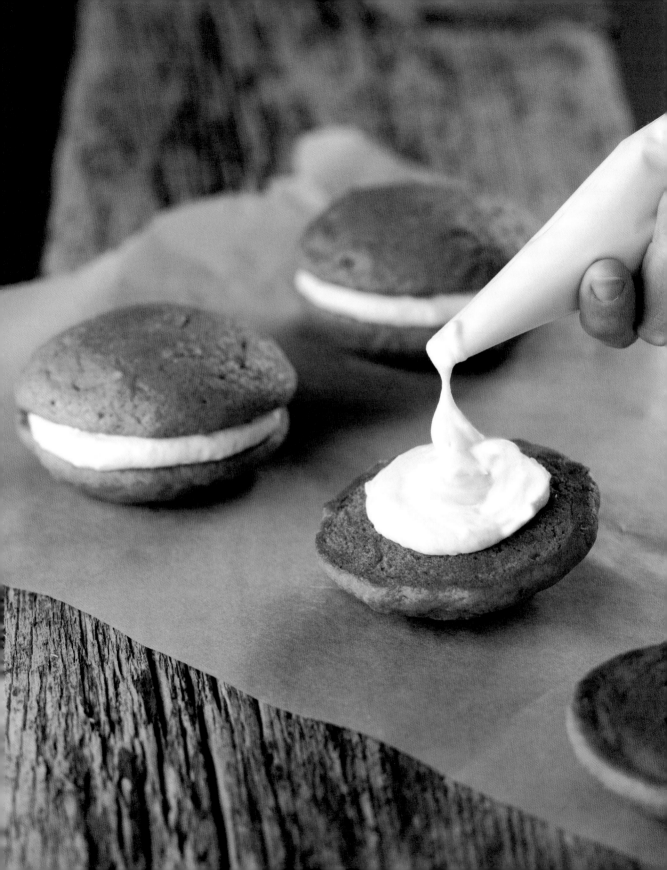

Maple-Pumpkin Moon Pies

In this comforting little cake, I combine warming spices and pumpkin with a creamy marshmallow filling.

Makes 12 servings

THC per serving: Please see page 54 to calculate.

Filling

2 cups powdered sugar, sifted
½ cup (8 tablespoons/1 stick) unsalted butter, slightly softened
1 (7-ounce) jar marshmallow creme (such as Fluff)
2 teaspoons maple extract

Cake

3 cups all-purpose flour
2 tablespoons ground cinnamon
1 teaspoon freshly grated nutmeg
¾ teaspoon ground cloves
1 tablespoon ground ginger
1½ teaspoons baking powder
1½ teaspoons baking soda
¾ teaspoon salt
6 tablespoons (¾ stick) unsalted butter, slightly softened
¾ cup firmly packed dark brown sugar
¼ cup Hey Sugar! (page 51)
½ cup granulated sugar
½ cup vegetable oil
1 tablespoon pure vanilla extract
3 large eggs
1 (15-ounce) can pure pumpkin puree
½ cup whole milk

1. Prepare the filling: In a large bowl using an electric mixer, beat together the powdered sugar and butter on medium speed until fluffy, about

2 minutes. Add the marshmallow creme and maple extract and beat until blended and smooth. Set aside.

2. Prepare the cake: Weigh the bowl that you will be using to hold the finished batter and write down this number.

3. In a separate large bowl, combine the flour, cinnamon, nutmeg, cloves, ginger, baking powder, baking soda, and salt. Set aside.

4. In the bowl you weighed previously, using an electric mixer, beat together the butter, brown sugar, Hey Sugar!, and granulated sugar on medium speed until light and fluffy. Gradually beat in the oil. Add the vanilla. Add the eggs one at a time, beating well after each addition. Beat in the pumpkin. Reduce the mixer speed to low and add half the flour mixture, then the milk, then the rest of the flour mixture, beating to blend between additions. Cover and refrigerate the batter for 1 hour.

5. Preheat the oven to 350°F. Arrange one rack in the bottom third of the oven and one rack in the top third of the oven. Line two baking sheets with parchment paper.

6. Weigh the batter, subtract the weight of the bowl, and divide by 24: This is your per-cake weight (2 cakes = 1 moon pie). Weigh out the batter for each cake and drop onto the prepared baking sheet, spacing them 2 inches apart.

7. Bake until the cakes are beginning to crack on top and a toothpick inserted into the centers comes out clean, 15 to 20 minutes. Let cool completely on the baking sheets on a wire rack. If you are going to freeze these, don't fill the cakes. Defrost and then fill.

8. Assemble the moon pies. When the cakes have cooled completely, spoon a large dollop of the filling (about 2 tablespoons) onto the flat side of half the cakes. Sandwich with the remaining cakes, pressing down slightly so that the filling spreads to the edges of the cake. Transfer to a baking sheet and cover with plastic wrap. Refrigerate for at least 30 minutes before serving.

9. Wrap tightly in aluminum foil and store in the refrigerator for up to 5 days, or in the freezer for up to 3 months.

CUPCAKES AND MUFFINS

DOUBLE CHOCOLATE-BANANA CUPCAKES
WITH FLUFFY COCONUT FROSTING · *144*

FRENCH TOAST CUPCAKES · *147*

KOOKY ADZUKI CUPCAKES · *151*

RUM RAISIN CUPCAKES · *155*

SHOT OF ESPRESSO MUFFINS · *158*

HOPS TO IT CUPCAKES · *160*

TWIX TRICKS CUPCAKES · *165*

Double Chocolate–Banana Cupcakes with Fluffy Coconut Frosting

There's nothing more intoxicating than the smell of cupcakes baking—except, of course, for the taste of cupcakes when you finally get to eat them! Your self-control will go out the window after a whiff of these deliciously desirable little cakes. The rich flavor of ripe bananas topped with fluffy frosting and a sprinkling of toasted, flaked coconut is pure decadence.

Makes 12 cupcakes

THC per serving: Please see page 54 to calculate.

Cupcakes

1¾ cups all-purpose flour
¼ cup unsweetened cocoa powder
1 teaspoon baking soda
¾ teaspoon baking powder
¼ teaspoon salt
2 very ripe large bananas
½ cup Buddha Budda (page 43), slightly softened
¾ cup sugar
2 large eggs
2 teaspoons pure vanilla extract
¼ cup buttermilk
½ cup mini chocolate chips

Frosting

1 cup sugar
2 tablespoons light corn syrup
3 tablespoons water
2 large egg whites
¼ teaspoon salt
1 teaspoon pure vanilla extract

1 cup unsweetened coconut flakes, lightly toasted

1. Prepare the cupcakes: Preheat the oven to 350°F. Line a 12-cup muffin tin with paper liners.

2. In a medium bowl, stir together the flour, cocoa powder, baking soda, baking powder, and salt. Set aside. In a small bowl, mash the bananas with a fork or potato masher. Set aside.

3. In a large bowl using an electric mixer, beat the Buddha Budda with the sugar on medium speed until creamy. Add the eggs one at a time, beating well after each addition. Add the mashed bananas, vanilla, and buttermilk and mix until just blended.

4. Reduce the mixer speed to low and add the flour mixture one-third at a time, beating until just blended. Fold in the chocolate chips.

5. Divide the batter evenly among the wells of the prepared muffin tin. Bake for 20 to 25 minutes, or until a toothpick inserted into the center of a muffin comes out clean. Let cool in the tin for 10 minutes, then transfer to a wire rack to cool completely.

6. Prepare the frosting: In a medium saucepan, combine the sugar, corn syrup, and the water. Heat over medium-high heat, stirring continuously, until the sugar has dissolved. Stop stirring and bring the mixture to a boil; keep at a boil for 2 minutes. Remove from the heat and set aside.

7. In a medium bowl using an electric mixer, beat the egg whites and salt on medium speed until frothy. Add the vanilla. Raise the mixer speed to high

and whip until soft peaks form. Slowly pour in the sugar syrup and beat until the mixture is glossy and holds stiff peaks.

8. Transfer the frosting to a piping bag fitted with the tip of your choice and frost the cupcakes, or simply frost them with a butter knife or small offset spatula. Sprinkle toasted coconut flakes over the top.

9. Store the frosted cupcakes in an airtight container in the refrigerator for up to 1 week. Unfrosted cupcakes can be stored in the freezer for up to 3 months.

French Toast Cupcakes

It's a cupcake made with bacon and maple syrup and cinnamon. Do you really need more convincing?

Makes 12 servings

THC per serving: Please see page 54 to calculate.

Topping

¼ **cup all-purpose flour**
¼ **cup sugar**
2½ **tablespoons unsalted butter, cut into ½-inch pieces and chilled**
½ **teaspoon ground cinnamon**
¼ **cup chopped pecans**

Cupcakes

1½ **cups all-purpose flour**
1 **cup sugar**
1½ **teaspoons baking powder**
1 **teaspoon ground cinnamon**
½ **teaspoon ground allspice**
¼ **teaspoon freshly grated nutmeg**
½ **teaspoon salt**
½ **cup Buddha Budda (page 43), slightly softened**
½ **cup sour cream**
2 **large eggs**
½ **teaspoon maple extract**
4 **slices bacon**

1. Prepare the topping: In a medium bowl, combine the flour, sugar, butter, cinnamon, and pecans. Using your fingers, mix in the butter until there are no pieces larger than a small pea. Cover and refrigerate until ready to use.

2. Prepare the cupcakes: Preheat the oven to 350°F. Line a 12-cup muffin tin with paper liners.

3. In a large bowl, whisk together the flour, sugar, baking powder, cinnamon, allspice, nutmeg, and salt. Set aside.

4. In a large bowl using an electric mixer, beat together the Buddha Budda, sour cream, eggs, and maple extract on medium speed until completely smooth. Reduce the mixer speed to low and add the flour mixture. Beat until just combined.

5. Fill each well of the muffin tin three-quarters of the way with batter. Divide the topping evenly and sprinkle it over the top of each cupcake, gently pressing it into the batter with your fingertips. Bake for 20 to 25 minutes, or until a toothpick inserted into the center of a cupcake comes out clean.

6. While the cupcakes are baking, cook the bacon according to the package directions. Transfer to a paper towel to absorb the excess oil and let cool.

7. Let the muffins cool in the tin for about 15 minutes, then transfer to a wire rack to cool completely. Cut the bacon into 12 pieces total and press a piece into the top of each muffin. Cupcakes can be stored in the freezer for up to 3 months. If you are going to freeze these, omit the bacon. Reheat in the toaster oven for extra deliciousness.

8. Store the bacon-topped cupcakes in an airtight container in the refrigerator for up to 1 week.

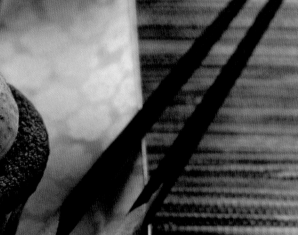

Kooky Adzuki Cupcakes

Dark chocolate and sweet adzuki topped with a richly flavored matcha frosting: delicious. Adzuki beans are a small red bean used in East Asian cuisine. When boiled with sugar or honey, they form a red paste that can be used in a variety of confections, from ice cream to glutinous rice cakes. Matcha is a finely milled green tea that tastes rich and earthy, with a lingering sweetness. East meets West!

Makes 12 cupcakes

THC per serving: Please see page 54 to calculate.

Adzuki Truffles
¾ cup red adzuki bean paste
¾ cup powdered sugar

Dark Chocolate Cupcakes
4 ounces unsweetened chocolate
1½ cups all-purpose flour
½ teaspoon baking soda
½ teaspoon salt
¾ cup coconut milk
1 teaspoon pure vanilla extract
½ cup Coconut Bliss (page 46), slightly softened
1 cup granulated sugar
2 large eggs

Matcha Green Tea Frosting
½ cup (8 tablespoons/1 stick) unsalted butter, slightly softened
4 ounces cream cheese
1½ cups powdered sugar
1 teaspoon matcha tea powder

1 tablespoon toasted sesame seeds, for garnish

1. Prepared the adzuki bean truffles: Combine the adzuki paste and powdered sugar in a small bowl and mix gently using your hands. Form the

mixture into 12 balls about 1 inch in diameter. Set them on a plate and cover with plastic wrap. Refrigerate or freeze while you are making the cupcakes.

2. Prepare the dark chocolate cupcakes: Preheat the oven to 350°F. Line a 12-cup muffin tin with paper liners.

3. Set up a double boiler with 2 to 3 inches of water in the bottom pot and bring the water to a simmer. Melt the unsweetened chocolate in the top section, stirring frequently until the chocolate is melted and smooth. Remove from the heat and set aside to cool slightly.

4. In a medium bowl, sift together the flour, baking soda, and salt. Set aside. In a small bowl, combine the coconut milk and vanilla. Set aside.

5. In a large bowl using an electric mixer, beat together the Coconut Bliss and granulated sugar on medium speed until light and fluffy, about 3 minutes. Mix in the melted chocolate. Add the eggs one at a time, beating for 30 seconds after each addition. Reduce the mixer speed to low and add about one-third of the flour mixture, beating just to combine. Add half of the coconut milk mixture and beat until just incorporated. Repeat with half the remaining flour, alternating between the dry and liquid mixtures; finish with the dry.

6. Fill each well of the muffin tin halfway with the batter (you'll use about half the batter). Place an adzuki bean truffle in the center of each well, pushing them down slightly. Divide the remaining batter evenly among the wells, making sure the adzuki truffles are completely covered.

7. Bake for 20 to 25 minutes or until a toothpick inserted near the edge of a cupcake comes out clean. Let cool completely in the pan. Transfer to a wire rack.

8. Prepare the matcha green tea frosting: In a medium bowl using an electric mixer, beat together the butter and cream cheese on medium speed until creamy.

9. Sift the powdered sugar and matcha powder into the cream cheese mixture and beat until smooth and creamy.

10. Transfer the frosting to a piping bag fitted with the tip of your choice and frost the cupcakes, or simply frost them with a butter knife or small offset spatula. Sprinkle with toasted sesame seeds.

11. Store the frosted cupcakes in an airtight container in the refrigerator for up to 1 week. Unfrosted cupcakes can be stored in the freezer for up to 3 months.

To make these cupcakes dairy-free, substitute this next frosting for the Matcha Green Tea Frosting:

Coconut Cream Frosting

1 (15-ounce) can coconut milk

2 teaspoons honey

½ teaspoon pure vanilla extract

1 teaspoon matcha tea powder

1. Place the can of coconut milk in the fridge overnight. This will allow the milk and the cream to separate.

2. Turn the can upside down and open it. Pour off the thin liquid, discarding it or reserving it for another use, and scoop the thick cream into a medium bowl.

3. Add the honey and vanilla to the coconut cream.

4. Using an electric mixer, whip the coconut cream on medium-high speed until fluffy. Beat in the matcha powder. Frost the cupcakes as directed.

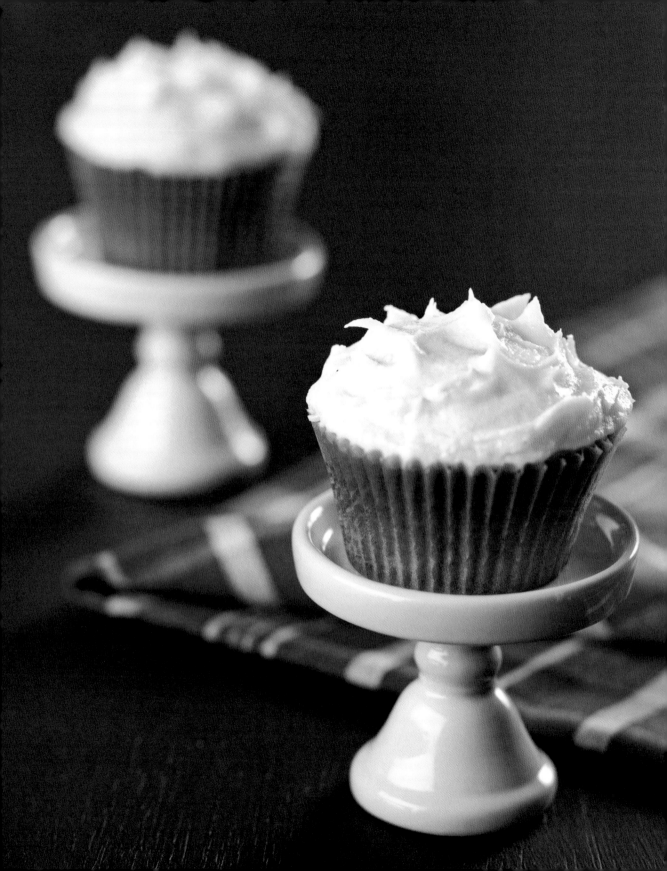

Rum Raisin Cupcakes

··

A sweet, grown-up cupcake with sophisticated flavors, this is more cosmopolitan than kid and may be just the ticket when the munchies strike during The Tonight Show Starring Jimmy Fallon. *Rum-soaked raisins, zesty spices, and sweet cream frosting all come together here, proving that ice cream isn't the only rum raisin treat. YUM!*

Makes 12 cupcakes

THC per serving: Please see page 54 to calculate.

Rum Raisins
¼ cup dark rum
½ cup golden raisins

Cupcakes
1 cup all-purpose flour
1¼ teaspoons baking powder
¼ teaspoon ground cinnamon
⅛ teaspoon ground allspice
⅛ teaspoon freshly grated nutmeg
½ cup Buddha Budda (page 43), slightly softened
2 tablespoons unsalted butter, slightly softened
¾ cup firmly packed light brown sugar
3 large eggs
1 tablespoon pure vanilla extract
¼ teaspoon pure rum extract

Sweet Cream Frosting
¼ cup (4 tablespoons/½ stick) unsalted butter, slightly softened
¼ cup heavy cream
2 cups powdered sugar, sifted
⅛ teaspoon salt

1. Prepare the rum raisins: In a small saucepan, warm the rum over low heat. Stir in the raisins and remove from the heat. Pour into a glass bowl, cover tightly with plastic wrap, and let sit at room temperature for at least 6 hours or overnight.

2. Prepare the cupcakes: Preheat the oven to 350°F. Line a 12-cup muffin tin with paper liners.

3. In a medium bowl, stir together the flour, baking powder, cinnamon, allspice, and nutmeg. Set aside.

4. In a large bowl using an electric mixer, beat together the Buddha Budda, butter, and brown sugar on medium speed until light and fluffy. Add the eggs one at a time, beating well after each addition.

5. Beat in the vanilla and rum extracts. Reduce the speed mixer to low, add the flour mixture, and mix until just combined. Fold in the rum raisins and any remaining liquid.

6. Divide the batter evenly among the wells of the prepared muffin tin. Bake for 20 to 25 minutes, or until golden brown and a toothpick inserted into the center of a cupcake comes out clean. Let cool in the tin for 5 minutes, then transfer to a wire rack to cool completely. Unfrosted cupcakes can be stored in the freezer for up to 3 months.

7. Prepare the sweet cream frosting: In a medium bowl using an electric mixer, beat the butter on medium speed until creamy. Reduce the mixer speed to low and add the cream and 1 cup of the powdered sugar; beat until well combined. Slowly add the remaining 1 cup sugar and the salt.

8. Transfer the frosting to a piping bag fitted with the tip of your choice and frost the cupcakes, or simply frost them with a butter knife or small offset spatula.

9. Store the frosted cupcakes in an airtight container in the refrigerator for up to 1 week.

Shot of Espresso Muffins

··

In this wonderfully ambrosial muffin, you'll combine the creamy flavor of white chocolate, the bitter edginess of espresso, and just the right amount of rich semi-sweet chocolate. Be prepared—you may find yourself wanting to tiptoe back into the kitchen for "just one more."

Makes 12 muffins

THC per serving: Please see page 54 to calculate.

Topping
6 tablespoons all-purpose flour
1½ teaspoons ground cinnamon
2 tablespoons firmly packed light brown sugar
2 tablespoons granulated sugar
3 tablespoons unsalted butter, cut into ½-inch pieces
½ cup pecans, chopped

Muffins
1 tablespoon finely ground espresso beans
1¾ cups all-purpose flour
1½ teaspoons baking powder
½ teaspoon salt
2 teaspoons ground cinnamon
½ teaspoon freshly grated nutmeg
¼ cup Hey Sugar! (page 51)
2 tablespoons granulated sugar
¼ cup white chocolate chips
½ cup semisweet chocolate chips
5 tablespoons unsalted butter, melted
2 tablespoons firmly packed light brown sugar
2 large eggs
½ cup milk
1 tablespoon pure vanilla extract

1. Preheat the oven to 375°F. Line a 12-cup muffin tin with paper liners.

2. Prepare the topping. In the bowl of a food processor, combine the flour, cinnamon, and brown and granulated sugars; pulse to combine. Add the butter and pecans and pulse until just crumbly. Do not overprocess. Set aside.

3. Prepare the muffins: In a large bowl, stir together the espresso, flour, baking powder, salt, cinnamon, nutmeg, Hey Sugar!, and granulated sugar. Place 1 tablespoon of this mixture in a small bowl and add the white and semisweet chocolate chips; toss to coat. (This helps keep the chips from sinking to the bottom of the muffins.) Set aside the remaining flour mixture.

4. In a large bowl using an electric mixer, combine the melted butter, brown sugar, eggs, vanilla, and milk on low speed. Add the flour mixture and beat to combine. Do not overbeat. Fold in the chips.

5. Divide the batter evenly among the wells of the prepared muffin tin. Evenly divide the topping and sprinkle onto the top of each muffin, gently pressing it into the batter with your fingertips. The muffin cups should be filled to the rim.

6. Bake for 15 to 20 minutes, or until a toothpick inserted into the center of a muffin comes out with a few moist crumbs clinging to it. Let cool in the tin for 10 minutes, then transfer to a wire rack and let cool completely.

7. Store the muffins in an airtight container in the refrigerator for up to 1 week, or in the freezer for up to 3 months.

Hops to It Cupcakes

Playful, rich, and just a tiny bit naughty, this is a cupcake with benefits. It's tender, spicy, and rich with the flavors of porter, coffee, and dark chocolate—the porter adds a toasty, caramelly touch. (I use Boulder Beer "Shake" Chocolate Porter in the recipe, but any porter beer or stout will work.) Fluffy orange filling and frosting cool the whole thing down.

The difference between stout and porter: Stout is roasted barley–centric, which gives a coffee-to-espresso aroma and flavor, while porter is more chocolate-and-mocha-oriented.

Makes 12 cupcakes

THC per serving: Please see page 54 to calculate.

Cupcakes

3 ounces unsweetened chocolate

½ cup Buddha Budda (page 43)

1½ cups cake flour (not self-rising)

¾ teaspoon baking soda

¼ teaspoon salt

1 teaspoon cayenne pepper

1 teaspoon ground cinnamon

2 tablespoons coarsely ground coffee beans

½ cup granulated sugar

½ cup firmly packed dark brown sugar

2 large eggs

⅓ cup plain Greek yogurt

1 teaspoon pure vanilla extract

¾ cup porter beer or stout beer

Orange Buttercream Filling and Frosting

3¾ cups powdered sugar

¾ cup (12 tablespoons/1½ sticks) unsalted butter, slightly softened

Zest of 1 medium orange

Ground cinnamon, for dusting

2 teaspoons pure vanilla extract

2 to 4 tablespoons fresh orange juice

1. Prepare the cupcakes: Preheat the oven to 350°F. Line a 12-cup muffin tin with paper liners.

2. In a medium saucepan, melt the unsweetened chocolate and Buddha Budda over low heat, stirring frequently, until the mixture is melted and smooth. Set aside to cool slightly.

3. In a large bowl, combine the flour, baking soda, salt, cayenne, cinnamon, and ground coffee. Set aside.

4. In a large bowl using an electric mixer, beat together the melted chocolate mixture and granulated and brown sugars on medium speed until well blended. Add the eggs one at a time, beating well after each addition. Add the yogurt and vanilla and continue beating until the color of the batter lightens slightly, 1 to 2 minutes.

5. Reduce the mixer speed to low and add half of the flour mixture. Beat until just combined. Mix in the porter, then add the remaining flour mixture and beat until just blended.

6. Carefully spoon the batter into the wells of the muffin tin, filling them about three-quarters full. Bake for 13 to 15 minutes, or until a toothpick inserted into the center of a cupcake comes out clean.

7. Let the cupcakes cool in the tin for 15 minutes, then transfer to a wire rack to cool completely. If you are going to freeze these, don't fill or frost them. Defrost them completely before filling and frosting.

8. Prepare the orange buttercream filling and frosting: In a large bowl using an electric mixer, cream together the powdered sugar, butter, orange zest, and vanilla on medium speed until well combined Add 2 tablespoons of the orange juice and beat until fluffy, adding more orange juice, if needed, to

create a spreadable consistency. Transfer the frosting to a piping bag fitted with a plain tip.

9. When the cupcakes are completely cooled, insert the tip of the piping bag into a cupcake and squeeze in the filling until you feel it push back a little bit. Repeat until all of the cupcakes have been filled.

10. Frost the cupcakes with the remaining buttercream from the piping bag, or simply frost them with a butter knife or small offset spatula. Dust the buttercream with a sprinkling of cinnamon.

11. Store in an airtight container in the refrigerator for up to 1 week, or freeze for up to 3 months.

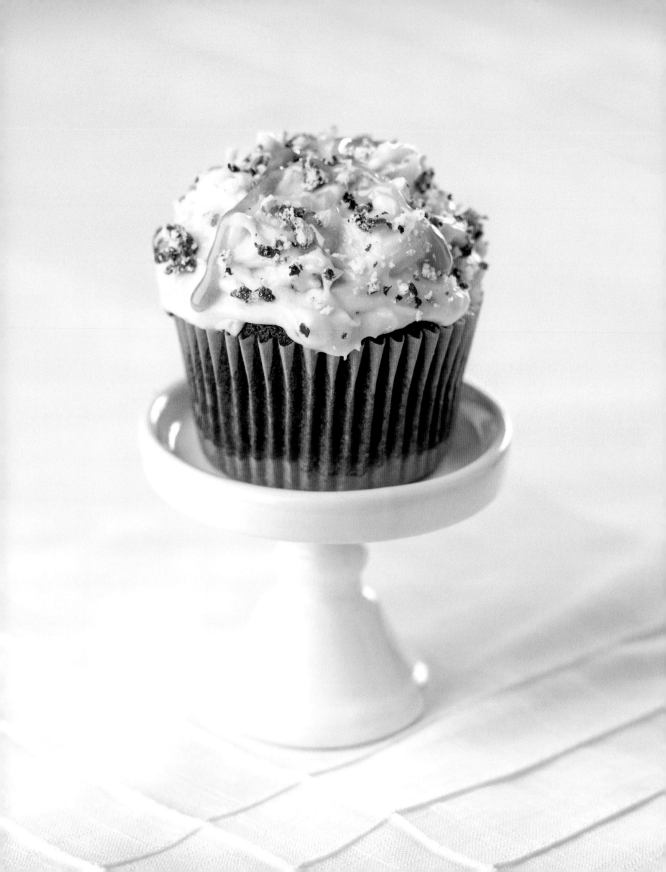

Twix Tricks Cupcakes

I haven't met a person yet who doesn't like Twix candy bars, but maybe people like that do exist. If so, this cupcake will change their minds. Give it a shot and see what you think.

Note: For high-altitude bakers, reduce the sugar in these cupcakes by 2 tablespoons and increase the flour by 3 tablespoons.

Makes 12 cupcakes

THC per serving: Please see page 54 to calculate.

Crust
1 cup Nilla wafers, broken into pieces
2 tablespoons unsalted butter, melted
¾ teaspoon granulated sugar

Chocolate Cupcakes
1 cup all-purpose flour
6 tablespoons unsweetened cocoa powder
¾ teaspoon baking powder
¾ teaspoon baking soda
½ teaspoon salt

½ cup Buddha Budda (page 43), slightly softened
1 cup granulated sugar
1 large egg
½ cup whole milk
1 tablespoon pure vanilla extract
¼ cup boiling water

Caramel Buttercream Frosting
½ cup (8 tablespoons/1 stick) unsalted butter, slightly softened
2 to 3 cups powdered sugar
¼ teaspoon salt

1 tablespoon pure vanilla extract
2 tablespoons whole milk
2 tablespoons jarred caramel sauce, warmed

2 to 3 mini Twix candy bars, crushed

1. Preheat the oven to 350°F. Line a 12-cup muffin tin with paper liners.

2. Prepare the crust: In the bowl of a food processor, combine the Nilla wafers, butter, and granulated sugar and pulse until well blended and fine crumbs form. Using your fingers, press 1 tablespoon of the crumbs evenly into the bottom of each lined well of the muffin tin. Bake for 3 to 5 minutes, or until the crust is just starting to turn light golden brown. Remove from the oven (leave the oven on).

3. Prepare the chocolate cupcakes: In a medium bowl, stir together the flour, cocoa powder, baking powder, baking soda, and salt. Set aside.

4. In a large bowl using an electric mixer, cream together the Buddha Budda and granulated sugar on medium speed until light and fluffy. Add the egg, milk, and vanilla and beat until well blended. Add the boiling water. Add the flour mixture, blending until just combined.

5. Divide the batter evenly among the wells of the muffin tin, pouring it over the baked crusts. Bake for 22 to 25 minutes, until a toothpick inserted into the center comes out clean. Transfer to a wire rack and let cool completely.

6. Prepare the caramel buttercream frosting: In a large bowl using an electric mixer, beat the butter on medium speed until smooth and creamy. Reduce the mixer speed to low and add the powdered sugar, salt, vanilla, milk, and caramel sauce. Raise the mixer speed to high and beat until light and fluffy.

7. Transfer the frosting to a piping bag fitted with the tip of your choice and frost the cupcakes, or simply frost them with a butter knife or a small offset spatula. Sprinkle the frosting with the crushed Twix bars. If you are going to freeze these, do not frost them.

8. Store in an airtight container in the refrigerator for up to 3 days, or freeze for up to 3 months.

TARTS AND PASTRIES

ROSEWATER BAKLAVA · *170*

BLUEBERRY-PEACH COBBLER · *173*

FOUR-AND-TWENTY APPLE PIE · *175*

POT TARTS · *179*

QUEEN OF TARTS · *183*

SWEETIE PIE PEAR TART · *187*

Rosewater Baklava

In this delicious, innovative take on baklava, you'll pile layer upon layer of heady goodness, filled with walnuts and pistachios, and infused with a splash of rosewater for an incredible flavor boost. Prepare for oohs, ahhs, and encores.

Makes 12 servings

THC per serving: Please see page 54 to calculate.

Rose Syrup
1⅓ cups sugar
⅔ cup honey
2 cinnamon sticks
8 (2 x ½-inch) strips orange peel
1½ cups water
2 teaspoons rosewater (see Notes, page 172)

Filling
2 cups coarsely chopped walnuts
1 cup coarsely chopped pistachios
1 teaspoon ground cinnamon
½ teaspoon ground cloves
⅓ cup sugar
½ cup (8 tablespoons/1 stick) unsalted butter
½ cup Buddha Budda (page 43)
1 pound (about 24 sheets) phyllo dough (see Notes, page 172)

1. Prepare the rose syrup: In a saucepan, combine the sugar, honey, cinnamon sticks, orange peel, and 1½ cups water and heat over medium heat until the sugar has dissolved. Raise the heat to high and bring the mixture to a boil. Remove from the heat. Stir in the rosewater. Transfer to a bowl, cover, and refrigerate until cold.

2. Preheat the oven to 325°F.

3. Prepare the filling: In a medium bowl, mix together the walnuts, pistachios, cinnamon, cloves, and sugar. Set aside.

4. In a small saucepan, melt together the unsalted butter and Buddha Budda over medium-low heat. Brush a 13 x 9 x 2-inch metal baking pan with some of the melted butter mixture.

5. Place one sheet of phyllo in the prepared pan. Brush with the melted butter mixture. Repeat with 7 more sheets, brushing the top of each with the melted butter before adding the next sheet. Keep the remaining dough covered with a damp towel while you work to keep it from drying out.

6. Sprinkle half of the nut mixture over the eighth sheet of buttered phyllo in the pan. Top with another sheet of phyllo and brush with the melted butter. Repeat with 7 more sheets, brushing the top of each with melted butter. Sprinkle the remaining nut mixture on top.

7. Finish layering the remaining 8 sheets of phyllo, brushing the top of each with the melted butter.

8. Using a sharp knife, make five diagonal cuts across the phyllo, cutting through the top layers only and spacing the cuts evenly. Repeat in the opposite direction to form a diamond pattern. Bake until golden brown, about 40 minutes.

9. Strain the chilled rose syrup. Spoon 1 cup of the syrup over the hot baklava; cover and refrigerate the remaining syrup. Recut the baklava along the lines, cutting all the way through the layers. Let stand for 4 hours. (The baklava can be made 1 day ahead. Cover and let stand at room temperature until ready to serve.) Serve with the remaining syrup poured over the top.

10. Wrap tightly in aluminum foil and store at room temperature for up to 5 days. To freeze, tightly wrap the baking pan of baklava first in a double layer of plastic wrap, then in a double layer of foil. Freeze for up to 3 months and thaw to room temperature before serving.

Notes: *Rosewater is available at Middle Eastern markets and specialty food stores.*

If the phyllo dough is frozen, thaw in the refrigerator overnight.

Blueberry-Peach Cobbler

I love this cobbler for dessert, hot out of the oven and topped with a mountain of unsweetened whipped cream. I love it just as much the next morning, served cold for breakfast (it's delicious alongside bacon and eggs). Feel free to substitute frozen blueberries and peaches if you can't find them fresh.

Makes 8 servings

THC per serving: Please see page 54 to calculate.

¼ cup (4 tablespoons/½ stick) unsalted butter, melted,
    plus more for the pan
4 cups sliced peeled peaches
2 pints blueberries (about 4 cups)
1 tablespoon cornstarch
1 teaspoon ground cinnamon
½ teaspoon ground ginger
¾ cup granulated sugar
2 tablespoons plus 2 teaspoons Hey Sugar! (page 51)
1 cup all-purpose flour
2 teaspoons baking powder
⅛ teaspoon freshly grated nutmeg
⅛ teaspoon salt
1 cup whole milk
Whipped cream, vanilla ice cream,
    or crème fraîche, for serving

1. Preheat the oven to 350°F. Lightly butter a 3-quart baking dish.

2. In a large bowl, combine the melted butter, peaches, blueberries, cornstarch, cinnamon, ginger, and ¼ cup of the granulated sugar.

3. In a medium bowl, whisk together the remaining ½ cup granulated sugar, the Hey Sugar!, flour, baking powder, nutmeg, and salt. Slowly whisk in the

milk. Pour the batter into the prepared baking dish and top with the fruit mixture. Bake for 45 to 50 minutes, until golden brown and the filling is bubbling and thick around the edges.

4. Serve hot from the oven topped with whipped cream, vanilla ice cream, or crème fraîche. Cover and refrigerate any leftover cobbler for up to 4 days.

Four-and-Twenty Apple Pie

Remember the nursery rhyme? Now that you're all grown up, it's time to bake the pie. This is a glorious fall dessert that sparkles with the bright flavors of apples and cinnamon. A nut-filled crumb topping finishes it off. Serve slices soon after the pie has cooled, with whipped cream or a scoop of your favorite ice cream. You can also have it straight from the fridge the next morning. Delicious with a cup of good hot coffee!

Makes 12 slices

THC per serving: Please see page 54 to calculate.

Crust

1⅔ cups all-purpose flour

¾ teaspoon salt

¾ teaspoon granulated sugar

½ cup plus 3 tablespoons unsalted butter, cut into small pieces and chilled

¼ to ⅓ cup ice water

Crumb Topping

½ cup firmly packed light brown sugar

½ cup granulated sugar

½ cup all-purpose flour

1 teaspoon ground cinnamon

¼ teaspoon salt

½ cup (8 tablespoons/1 stick) unsalted butter, cut into small pieces and chilled

1 cup walnuts, coarsely chopped

Filling

¾ cup granulated sugar

¼ cup Hey Sugar! (page 51)

½ cup all-purpose flour

1 teaspoon ground cinnamon

⅛ teaspoon salt

16 ounces sour cream

2 large eggs, lightly beaten

2 teaspoons pure vanilla extract

6 Granny Smith apples (about 2½ pounds), peeled, cored, and cut into ¼-inch wedges

1. Prepare the crust: In the bowl of a food processor, combine the flour, salt, and granulated sugar and pulse to blend. Add the butter and pulse until pea-size pieces form. With the machine running, add the water, 1 tablespoon at a time, until the mixture just comes together.

2. Press the dough into a 10-inch springform pan. Refrigerate until firm, about 1 hour.

3. Preheat the oven to 450°F. Place a rimmed baking sheet on the lowest oven rack (this is to catch any drips as the pie bakes).

4. Prepare the crumb topping: In a large bowl, whisk together the brown and granulated sugars, flour, cinnamon, and salt. Cut in the butter with a fork or pastry cutter. Fold in the walnuts. Press the mixture into large clumps with your hands. Cover and refrigerate until ready to use.

5. Prepare the filling: In a large bowl, whisk together the granulated sugar, Hey Sugar!, flour, cinnamon, and salt; combine well. Stir in the sour cream, eggs, and vanilla until thoroughly combined. Add the apples and toss to coat well. Pour the apple mixture into the chilled crust.

6. Bake the pie for 10 minutes. Reduce the oven temperature to 350°F and bake until the apples are golden brown, the juices are bubbling, and the crust is golden brown, about 45 minutes.

7. Remove the topping from the refrigerator and crumble it over the hot apple filling. Bake until the topping is browned and set, the apples are ten-

der, and the bottom crust is thoroughly baked, about 50 minutes. Let cool completely on a wire rack, 3 to 4 hours.

8. Run a knife around the edge of the pan to loosen the crust and remove the outside ring of the springform pan before slicing and serving. Refrigerate any leftover pie, covered, for up to 4 days.

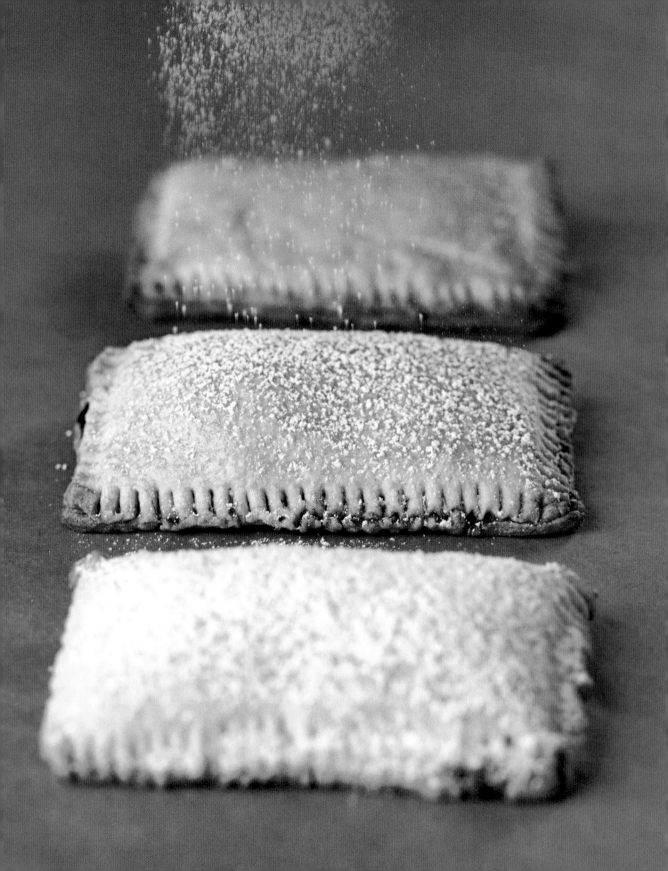

Pot Tarts

These little pillows of pastry brimming with a sweet or savory filling will satisfy your soul. Serve them warm from the oven, or gently reheat in a toaster oven.

Makes 9 tarts

THC per serving: Please see page 54 to calculate.

2 cups all-purpose flour, plus more for dusting
2 tablespoons Hey Sugar! (page 51)
1 teaspoon salt
1 cup (2 sticks) chilled unsalted butter, cut into pieces
2 large eggs
2 tablespoons whole milk
Fillings (see pages 180–181)
Raw sugar and powdered sugar, for dusting sweet tarts (optional)
Sesame seeds, poppy seeds, or coarse salt, for sprinkling savory tarts (optional)

1. Line a baking sheet with parchment paper.

2. In the bowl of a food processor, combine the flour, Hey Sugar!, and salt. Add the butter and pulse until it forms pea-size pieces, 1 to 2 minutes.

3. In a small bowl, whisk together one of the eggs and the milk. While pulsing, gradually pour the egg mixture through the top spout of the food processor; pulse just until the dough comes together.

4. Divide the dough in half. Place one piece on a lightly floured work surface and roll it into a 9 x 12-inch rectangle about ⅛ inch thick. Cut the dough sheet into nine 3 x 4-inch rectangles. Repeat with the second piece of dough so that you have a total of 18 rectangles.

5. Place 1 heaping tablespoon of the filling of your choice in the center of half the rectangles. Place the remaining rectangles on top of the filling-

covered rectangles, using your fingertips to press around the edges; seal by pressing the edges with the tines of a fork. Gently place the tarts on the prepared baking sheet.

6. Preheat the oven to 400°F.

7. In a small bowl, beat the remaining egg. Brush the entire surface of each tart with the beaten egg. Prick the top of each tart multiple times with a fork. If making sweet tarts, dust the tops with a sprinkling of raw sugar; if making savory tarts, sprinkle with sesame or poppy seeds or a light dusting of coarse salt. Refrigerate for 30 minutes.

8. Bake for 20 to 25 minutes, until the tarts are a light golden brown. Let cool on the baking sheet on a wire rack. If making sweet tarts, dust with a sprinkling of powdered sugar.

9. Wrap tightly in aluminum foil and store in the refrigerator for up to 5 days.

Sweet Pot Tarts

Jam
1 tablespoon cornstarch
1 tablespoon cold water
¾ cup of your favorite jam

Mix the cornstarch and water together in a small saucepan. Stir in the jam and blend well. Bring the mixture to a boil over medium heat and simmer, stirring, for 2 minutes. Remove from the heat and set aside to cool.

Cinnamon Cream Cheese
6 ounces cream cheese, slightly softened
3 tablespoons sugar
1 teaspoon ground cinnamon

In a medium bowl using an electric mixer, beat together the cream cheese, sugar, and cinnamon on high speed until smooth and creamy.

Savory Pot Tarts

Omit granulated sugar in the Pot Tarts dough (page 179), and skip the raw and powdered sugar topping.

Cheesy-Olive
3 ounces cream cheese, slightly softened
½ cup shredded cheddar cheese
1 tablespoon finely chopped assorted olives

In a medium bowl using an electric mixer, beat together the cream cheese, cheddar, and olives on medium-high speed until smooth and creamy.

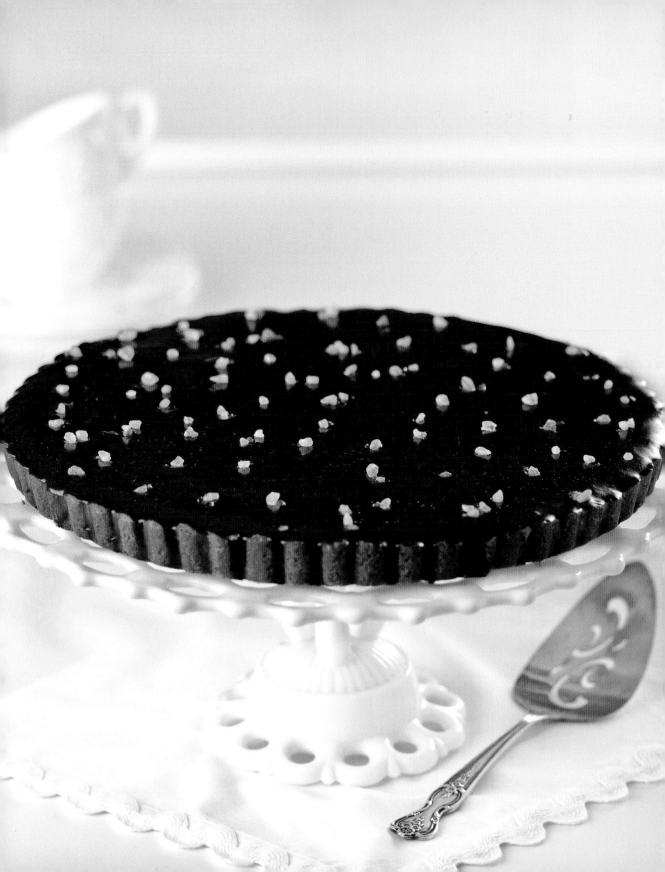

Queen of Tarts

· ·

This outrageously elegant tart combines copious amounts of dark chocolate with the sultry taste of almonds and a splash of rum. The intense flavor and silky texture stand up well to the crunch of Himalayan pink salt sprinkled over the top. What a fabulous way to get your chocolate fix! If you are sensitive to gluten, make sure your powdered sugar is labeled gluten-free.

Makes 8 servings

THC per serving: Please see page 54 to calculate.

Chocolate Pastry Dough

3 tablespoons unsalted butter, chilled, plus more for the pan

1 cup plus 3 tablespoons sifted powdered sugar

2⅓ cups almond flour

2½ tablespoons unsweetened cocoa powder

½ teaspoon fine sea salt

6 tablespoons Buddha Budda (page 43), chilled

1 large egg, lightly beaten

1 teaspoon pure vanilla extract

Almond Cream

½ cup (8 tablespoons/1 stick) unsalted butter, slightly softened

½ cup granulated sugar

1 large egg

1 cup finely ground blanched almonds

3 tablespoons dark rum

1 teaspoon pure almond extract

1 tablespoon almond flour

Chocolate Filling

7 ounces bittersweet chocolate, very finely chopped

2 teaspoons brewed espresso

3 tablespoons light corn syrup

1 cup heavy cream

3 tablespoons unsalted butter, slightly softened

1 teaspoon Himalayan pink salt, coarsely ground, or coarsely ground sea salt

1. Prepare the pastry dough: Butter a 10-inch tart pan with a removable bottom.

2. In the bowl of a food processor, combine the powdered sugar, almond flour, cocoa powder, and fine sea salt. Add the Buddha Budda and butter and pulse until the mixture resembles coarse sand. Add the egg and vanilla and pulse until dough just comes together. Press the dough evenly over the bottom and up the sides of the prepared tart pan. Cover with plastic wrap and refrigerate for at least 2 hours, or up to 3 days.

3. Preheat the oven to 375°F.

4. Prepare the almond cream: In a large bowl using an electric mixer, cream together the butter and granulated sugar on medium speed until light and fluffy. Add the egg, ground almonds, rum, almond extract, and almond flour and beat until smooth.

5. Remove the pastry from the refrigerator. Spoon the almond cream evenly over the crust. Bake until the almond cream is lightly browned and the pastry is crisp, about 10 minutes. Let cool in the tart pan on a wire rack. Once cool enough to handle, remove the outer ring from the tart pan and let cool completely. (Removing the ring allows the drizzled chocolate to drip down the sides, but it's fine to work with the ring on, if that's easier.)

6. Prepare the chocolate filling: In a medium bowl, combine the chocolate, espresso, and corn syrup. Place the heavy cream in a small saucepan and bring to a gentle simmer. Pour the cream over the chocolate mixture and gently stir until the chocolate has melted and the mixture is smooth. Add the butter and stir until it has melted.

7. Pour the chocolate filling over the almond cream. Pop any surface bubbles with a toothpick. Let sit for 15 minutes, then dust the top of the tart with a sprinkling of pink salt. Let the tart set, about 1 hour.

8. Serve, or store tightly wrapped in aluminum foil in the refrigerator for up to 3 days.

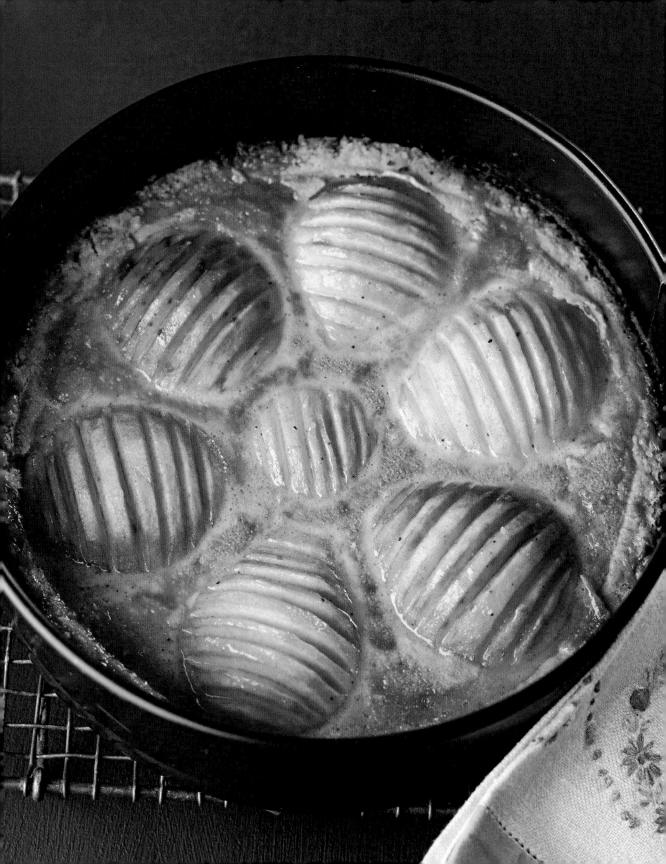

Sweetie Pie Pear Tart

....

In this recipe, tart meets soufflé and the two get along beautifully. I like to serve this enticing tart just as it is, filled with the incredible flavors of sweet pears, apricot jam, and vanilla. It's simplicity at its best.

Makes 8 servings

THC per serving: Please see page 54 to calculate.

Crust

½ cup (8 tablespoons/1 stick) unsalted butter, cut into pieces and chilled
1 tablespoon granulated sugar
1⅓ cups all-purpose flour
2 tablespoons slivered almonds
1 large egg

Filling

4 ripe small pears, such Anjou, Bosc, or Bartlett
2 large eggs
3 tablespoons Hey Sugar! (page 51)
¾ cup granulated sugar
2 tablespoons heavy cream
1 tablespoon unsalted butter, melted
1 teaspoon pure vanilla extract
¼ teaspoon freshly grated nutmeg
1 teaspoon lemon zest
3 tablespoons all-purpose flour

Glaze

½ cup apricot jam
1 tablespoon orange liqueur or water

1. Preheat the oven to 425°F.

2. Prepare the crust: In the bowl of a food processor, combine the butter, granulated sugar, flour, and almonds and pulse until crumbly. Add the egg

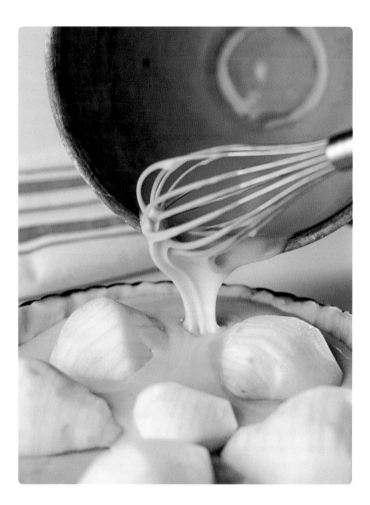

and pulse until the mixture forms a ball. Press the dough evenly over the bottom and up the sides of a 10-inch tart or springform pan. Chill the dough in the pan for 30 minutes.

3. Prepare the filling: Peel, halve, and core the pears. Place the pears, cut side down, on a cutting board. Using a sharp knife, evenly score lines horizontally across each pear half, about ⅛ inch deep and ¼ inch apart. Do not cut

through the pear. Arrange five to seven of the pear halves in the crust, with the narrow end of each pointing toward the center. Cut a freehand circle (it doesn't have to be perfect) from the remaining pear half and place it in the pie's center. (Feel free to eat the rest of that pear.)

4. In a medium bowl, beat the eggs until pale and thick. Add the Hey Sugar!, granulated sugar, heavy cream, melted butter, vanilla, nutmeg, lemon zest, and flour, and blend well. Pour the mixture over the pears. Bake for 10 to 15 minutes, then reduce the oven temperature to 400°F and bake for 20 to 25 minutes more, or until set and golden brown. Remove to a rack.

5. While the tart is baking, prepare the glaze: In a small saucepan, heat the jam over medium heat until melted. Stir in the liqueur. Press the mixture though a fine-mesh strainer into a bowl.

6. Brush the glaze over the top of the hot tart. Let cool, then remove the sides from the tart pan before slicing the tart into eight equal pieces. Refrigerate any leftover tart, well wrapped, for up to 4 days.

ICE CREAMS AND SORBETS

WICKED CHOCOLATE SORBET · *192*

COOL IT! COCONUT-VANILLA ICE CREAM · *193*

LAVENDER ICE CREAM · *197*

SWEET TEMPTATION MANGO SORBET · *201*

MIND ERASER PARFAITS · *202*

POP STAR PEANUT BUTTER PARFAIT · *205*

Wicked Chocolate Sorbet

....

Chiller instincts: This vanilla-kissed, dark-chocolate sorbet is intensely flavored but goes down easy. If you're in the mood for a truly wicked extravagance, I suggest ice cream sandwiches made with Lucie in the Sky cookies (page 103).

Makes 6 servings

THC per serving: Please see page 54 to calculate.

6 ounces bittersweet chocolate, finely chopped
¾ cup unsweetened cocoa powder
2¼ cups water
¾ cup plus 2 tablespoons granulated sugar
2 tablespoons Hey Sugar! (page 51)
1 tablespoon pure vanilla extract

1. Place the bittersweet chocolate and cocoa in a large saucepan. Slowly whisk in 1 cup water until the cocoa has dissolved and there are no lumps.

2. Whisk in the granulated sugar, Hey Sugar!, and remaining 1¼ cups water. Bring to a boil, stirring, over medium heat. Remove from the heat. Stir in the vanilla. Cover with plastic wrap and refrigerate overnight to thoroughly chill.

3. Pour the chilled sorbet base into the canister of an ice cream maker and process according to the manufacturer's directions. Remove the sorbet from the canister and place in an airtight container.

4. Store in the freezer for up to 3 months.

Cool It! Coconut-Vanilla Ice Cream

To come up with this recipe, I took a light, refreshing vanilla ice cream and fortified it with a strong hit of coconut. It makes a wonderful ice cream sandwich when paired with the Big S Oatmeal Cookie (sans filling, of course; page 115); or try it with Lucie in the Sky cookies (page 103). Remember to count the amount of THC you are using when making ice cream sandwiches—it adds up!

Makes 6 servings

THC per serving: Please see page 54 to calculate.

2 cups heavy cream
1 (15-ounce) can cream of coconut
¾ cup granulated sugar
2 tablespoons Hey Sugar! (page 51)
Pinch of salt
1 vanilla bean
6 large egg yolks

1. In a medium saucepan, combine the heavy cream, cream of coconut, granulated sugar, Hey Sugar!, and salt and heat over medium heat until the mixture just begins to simmer. Scrape the seeds from the vanilla bean into the mixture, cover, and remove from the heat. (If you like, you can save the vanilla pod and place it in a sugar canister.) Let steep for 30 minutes.

2. In a large bowl, beat the egg yolks until they lighten in color. While whisking continuously, add a ladleful of the warm cream mixture to the eggs to temper them. Continue whisking in the warm cream mixture until about one-third of the mixture has been added. Pour the tempered egg mixture back into the saucepan with the rest of the cream mixture and set the saucepan over medium-high heat. Cook, whisking continuously, until

the mixture thickens slightly and coats the back of a spoon (do not allow the mixture to come to a boil).

3. Pour the warmed custard through a fine-mesh sieve into a large bowl. Let cool. When cool, cover with plastic wrap and refrigerate overnight to thoroughly chill.

4. Pour the chilled custard into the canister of an ice cream maker and process according to the manufacturer's directions. Remove the ice cream from the canister and place in an airtight container.

5. Store in the freezer for up to 3 months.

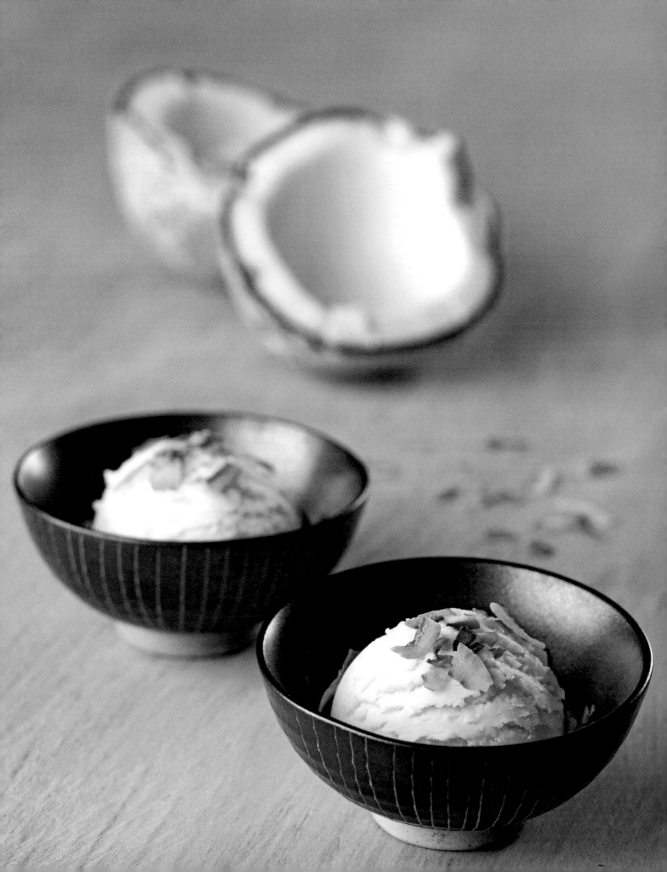

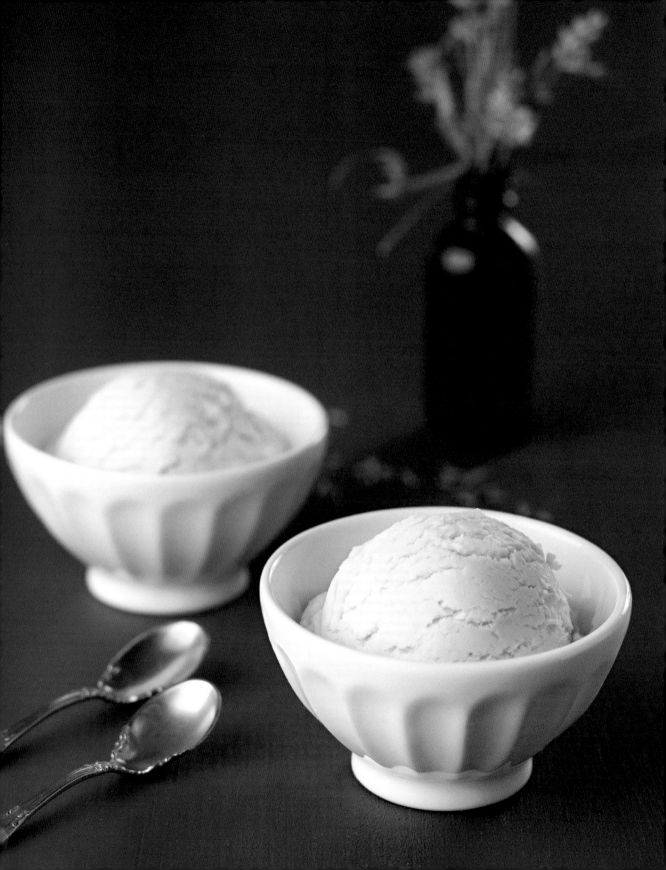

Lavender Ice Cream

· ·

This ice cream is simply delightful over warm peach pie, or scooped into a bowl and topped with Magic Moment Sauce (page 276), or in an ice cream sandwich using Feel the Love Lemon Sandwich Cookies (page 99). Take a cool, refreshing bite, and feel yourself relax.

Makes 6 servings

THC per serving: Please see page 54 to calculate.

2 cups whole milk

3 tablespoons dried organic culinary lavender (see Note, page 198)

5 large egg yolks

2 tablespoons Hey Sugar! (page 51)

½ cup plus 1 tablespoon granulated sugar

1 cup heavy cream

1. In a medium saucepan, combine the milk and the lavender. Bring to a simmer over medium heat, then cover and remove from the heat. Let steep for 6 minutes. Strain the mixture through a fine-mesh sieve into a bowl, discarding the lavender in the sieve.

2. In the bowl of an electric mixer, combine the egg yolks, Hey Sugar!, and granulated sugar. Beat on medium-high speed until very thick and pale yellow, 3 to 5 minutes. Meanwhile, return the milk to a medium saucepan and bring to a simmer over medium-low heat.

3. While whisking continuously, add a ladleful of the warm milk mixture to the egg yolk mixture to temper it. Continue whisking in the warm milk mixture until you have added half. Pour the tempered egg yolk mixture into the saucepan with the remaining milk. Cook over low heat, stirring continuously, until the mixture is thick enough to coat the back of a wooden spoon.

4. Remove from the heat and immediately stir in the cream. Pour the warmed custard through a fine-mesh sieve into a large bowl. Let cool, then cover with plastic wrap and refrigerate overnight to thoroughly chill.

5. Pour the chilled custard into the canister of an ice cream maker and process according to the manufacturer's directions. Remove the ice cream from the canister and place in an airtight container.

6. Store in the freezer for up to 3 months.

Note: *If you don't like lavender, you can change this recipe to vanilla by omitting the lavender and using the seeds scraped from one vanilla bean. If you make the vanilla version, do not strain the milk after simmering.*

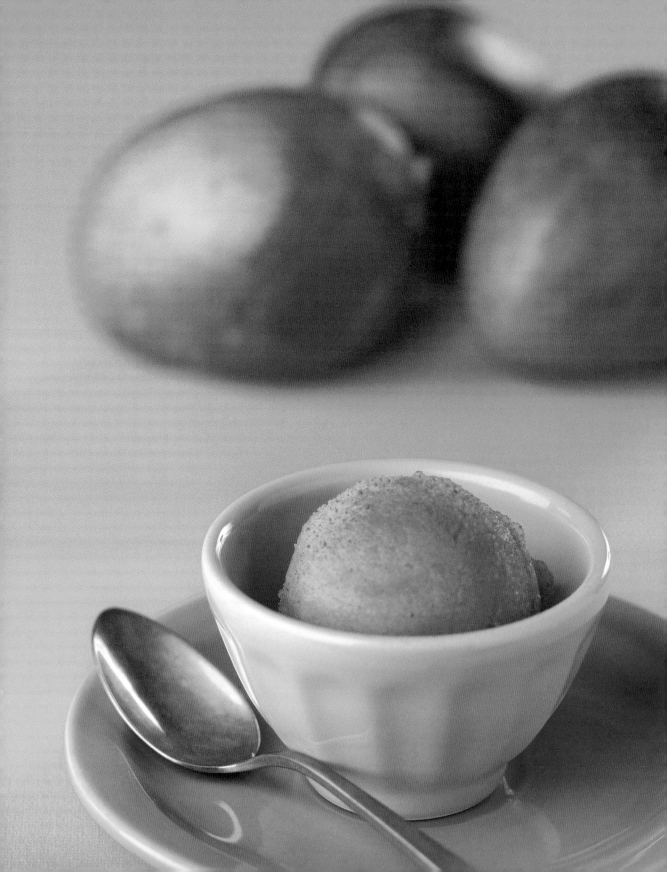

Sweet Temptation Mango Sorbet

Make this delicious sorbet recipe when you need a little Latin in your life. It's sweet and satisfying and tastes like Cinco de Mayo—the heat from the spices plays excitingly against the chill of the sorbet. I use a combination of ground chipotle and cayenne peppers, but you can try your favorites. I like it hot, so I use a full tablespoon of chili powder; if you prefer yours on the mild side, go with 1½ teaspoons.

Makes 6 servings

THC per serving: Please see page 54 to calculate.

4½ to 5 cups diced ripe mango
2 tablespoons plus 2 teaspoons Hey Sugar! (page 51)
½ cup plus 2 tablespoons granulated sugar
¼ cup fresh lime juice
1½ teaspoons to 1 tablespoon chili powder, plus more for serving
½ teaspoon coarse salt, plus more for serving

1. In the bowl of a food processor, combine the mango and ¼ cup water and process until smooth, about 30 seconds. Pour through a fine-mesh strainer into a large measuring cup, pushing the puree through the strainer with a spoon, until you have 3 cups of puree.

2. Transfer the strained puree to a large bowl and whisk in the Hey Sugar!, granulated sugar, lime juice, chili powder, and salt until well blended. Cover with plastic wrap and refrigerate overnight to thoroughly chill.

3. Pour the chilled sorbet base into the canister of an ice cream maker and process according to the manufacturer's directions. Remove the sorbet from the canister and place in an airtight container.

4. Serve with a sprinkling of chili powder and coarse salt. Store in the freezer for up to 3 months.

Mind Eraser Parfaits

I know this recipe looks complicated, but trust me, it's well worth all the time and energy you are going to put into it. This is one spoon-worthy dessert. (Of course, you can always make just the sorbet, or the ice cream, or the macaroons, or the hot fudge sauce, and eat that. Just sayin'.)

Be careful when you make this recipe, as it's combining several already infused recipes. Take note of the milligrams of THC you are adding to the total, and substitute your favorite ice cream, sorbets, cookies, or sauces for the infused ones if you don't want such a potent treat.

Makes 8 parfaits

THC per serving: Please see page 54 to calculate.

Wicked Chocolate Sorbet (page 192)
Cool It! Coconut-Vanilla Ice Cream (page 193)
½ cup Ecstasy Sauce (page 273)
1 cup heavy cream, whipped
1 tablespoon cacao nibs (optional)
French Kiss Toasted Macaroons (page 117)

1. Set out eight parfait glasses. Put one small scoop of Wicked Chocolate Sorbet into the bottom of each glass. Top with one small scoop of Cool It! Coconut-Vanilla Ice Cream and 1 tablespoon of Ecstasy Sauce.

2. Repeat the layering process once more. Top with a dollop of whipped cream, a sprinkling of cacao nibs, if using, and a French Kiss Toasted Macaroon. Serve immediately.

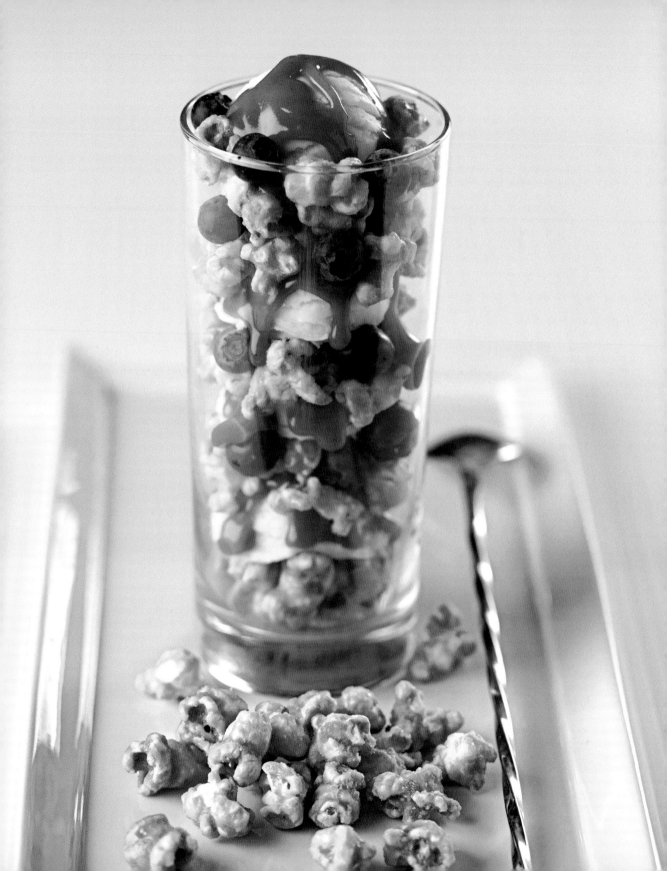

Pop Star Peanut Butter Parfait

Now, I know you may be thinking, Peanut butter, caramel, and blueberries, all in one dish? *But give it a chance. You'll find that a soft ice cream pillow drizzled with warm peanut butter sauce, all carried by crunchy, chewy caramel corn, with a few blueberries tossed in for good measure, is truly the ultimate dessert. Please make sure you watch the milligrams of THC you are adding when making a dessert like this one, which uses more than one infused recipe.*

I created Pop Star Peanut Butter Parfait on a warm July day. We had just finished making a particularly large batch of Pop Star for a customer, and there it was, cooling on the racks. The scent of caramel filled the kitchen. I knew I'd have extra and tried to think of what I might do with it. It's summer, I thought, ice cream season, and fresh, sweet blueberries are readily available, and we have plenty of peanut butter. So I prepared the ice cream base and went out to buy fresh blueberries. The next day, I made the ice cream and the peanut butter sauce. I spooned layers of each component into tall glasses. Everyone in the kitchen tried the parfait, and we all agreed that it was a crazy combination, but the flavors and textures blended gracefully—and deliciously.

Makes 1 serving

THC per serving: Please see page 54 to calculate.

2 small scoops vanilla ice cream or Cool It! Coconut-Vanilla Ice Cream (page 193)
2 tablespoons Silky Sweet Peanut Butter Sauce (page 275), warmed
2 tablespoons Pop Star Caramel Corn (page 246)
Fresh blueberries

To assemble the parfait, put one scoop of ice cream into the bottom of a parfait glass. Top with 1 tablespoon of the warmed peanut butter sauce and 1 tablespoon of the popcorn. Repeat the layering process once more, then top with a sprinkling of the fresh blueberries. Serve immediately.

PUDDINGS AND FLANS

LICK THE SPOON! BUTTERSCOTCH PUDDING · *209*

VANILLA ANGEL CRÈME BRÛLÉE · *211*

PUMPKIN FLAN WITH PUMPKIN SEED PRALINE · *214*

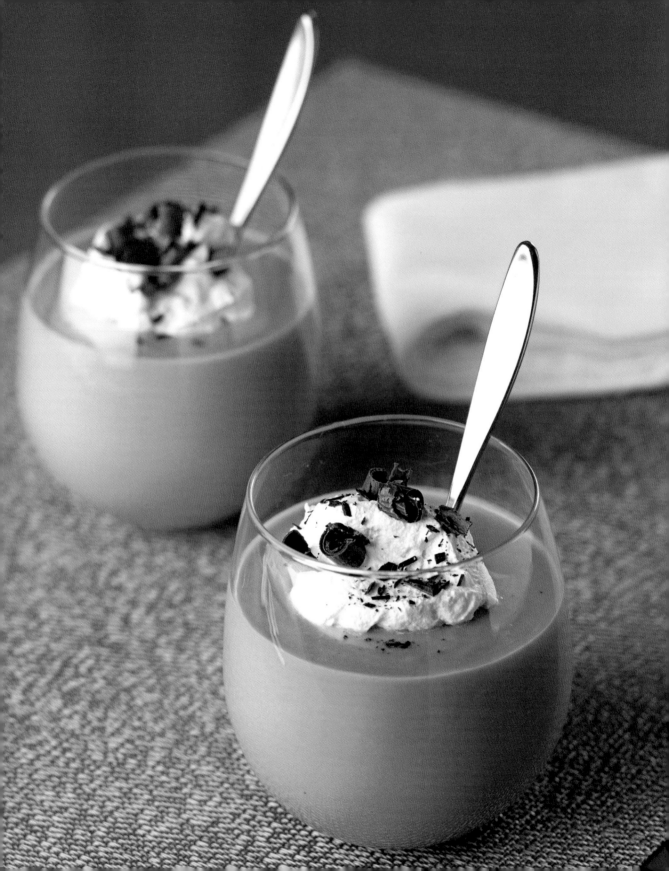

Lick the Spoon! Butterscotch Pudding

··

This velvety butterscotch concoction spiked with a touch of Scotch whiskey pays boozy homage to childhood puddings.

Makes 4 servings

THC per serving: Please see page 54 to calculate.

¼ cup (4 tablespoons/½ stick) salted butter
1 cup firmly packed dark brown sugar
1 tablespoon plus 1 teaspoon Hey Sugar! (page 51)
½ teaspoon coarse sea salt
3 tablespoons arrowroot powder
2½ cups whole milk
2 large eggs
½ cup butterscotch chips
2 teaspoons Scotch (any Scotch will do)
1 tablespoon pure vanilla extract
Unsweetened whipped cream, for serving
Chocolate shavings, for garnish

1. In a medium saucepan, melt the butter over medium heat. Add the brown sugar, Hey Sugar!, and salt; stir until well blended. Remove from the heat.

2. In a small bowl, whisk together the arrowroot powder and ¼ cup of the milk until smooth, then whisk in the eggs.

3. Gradually pour the remaining 2¼ cups of milk into the melted brown sugar mixture, whisking continuously, then whisk in the arrowroot mixture.

4. Return the pan to the stovetop over medium heat and bring the mixture to a boil, whisking continuously. Once it starts to bubble, reduce the heat to low and continue to cook at a gentle simmer, still whisking continuously,

until the pudding has thickened and coats the back of a spoon, 1 to 1½ minutes.

5. Remove from the heat and stir in the butterscotch chips, Scotch, and vanilla. If the mixture separates, continue stirring until it becomes smooth and creamy.

6. Divide the mixture evenly among four mugs or ramekins, cover, and refrigerate for at least 4 hours. Top with whipped cream and chocolate shavings.

Vanilla Angel Crème Brûlée

This creamy, dreamy, classic crème brûlée with a twist is topped with sparkly cara-melized sugar. Plus, you get to use a torch! How fun is that?!

Makes 4 servings

THC per serving: Please see page 54 to calculate.

Custard

2 cups heavy cream
2 tablespoons plus 2 teaspoons Hey Sugar! (page 51)
½ cup plus 1 tablespoon granulated sugar
1 vanilla bean, split lengthwise
4 large egg yolks
¼ teaspoon coarse salt

Topping

3 tablespoons granulated sugar
3 tablespoons brown sugar

1. Preheat the oven to 300°F. Place four 5-ounce baking dishes in a large roasting pan. Bring a pot of water to a boil.

2. Prepare the custard: In a medium saucepan, combine the cream, Hey Sugar!, and ¼ cup of the granulated sugar. Scrape the vanilla bean seeds into the saucepan, then add the pod. Heat over medium heat just until the mixture starts to bubble around the edges, 7 to 8 minutes (do not let boil).

3. In a large bowl, whisk the egg yolks with the remaining granulated sugar and the salt.

4. While whisking continuously, add a ladleful of the hot cream mixture to the egg yolk mixture to temper it. One at a time, whisk in two more ladles of

the hot cream mixture, whisking well after each addition. Gradually whisk in the remaining cream mixture. Strain the mixture through a fine-mesh sieve into a large liquid measuring cup.

5. Divide the custard evenly among the baking dishes in the roasting pan. Pour enough boiling water into the roasting pan to come halfway up the sides of the dishes. Bake until the custards are just set (they should tremble slightly in the center when shaken), 35 to 45 minutes.

6. Remove the pan from the oven. Let cool for 10 minutes, then carefully remove the dishes from the hot water bath and let cool on a wire rack for 30 minutes. Cover with plastic wrap and refrigerate for at least 2 hours, or up to 3 days.

7. Remove the crème brûlées from the refrigerator and let sit at room temperature for at least 30 minutes.

8. Prepare the topping: Combine the granulated and brown sugars in a small bowl. Sprinkle 1½ tablespoons of the sugar mixture on top of each custard.

9. Caramelize the tops by passing the flame of a kitchen torch in a circular motion 1 to 2 inches above the surface of each custard until the sugar bubbles, turns amber, and forms a crispy surface. If you don't have a torch, place the ramekins under the broiler until the sugar melts, about 2 minutes. Watch carefully to make sure they do not burn. Serve immediately.

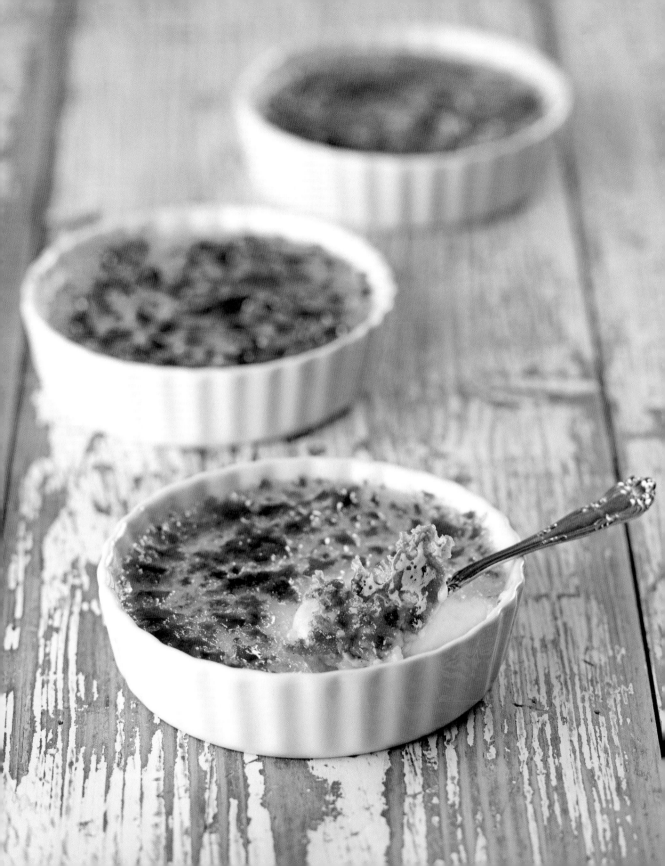

Pumpkin Flan with Pumpkin Seed Praline

....

Smooth and straightforward, with big, vibrant flavors, topped with shards of crunchy pumpkin seed praline—each bite of this delicious flan is a decadent treat.

Makes 8 servings

THC per serving: Please see page 54 to calculate.

1¾ cups granulated sugar
1 cup whole milk
2 (5-ounce) cans evaporated milk
2 tablespoons plus 2 teaspoons Hey Sugar! (page 51)
5 large eggs
¼ teaspoon salt
1¾ cups pure pumpkin puree
2 tablespoons tequila
1 tablespoon orange zest
2 teaspoons ground cinnamon
1 teaspoon ground ginger
¼ teaspoon ground cardamom
¼ teaspoon freshly grated nutmeg
1 tablespoon pure vanilla extract

Pumpkin Seed Praline
Vegetable oil, for greasing the foil
1 cup granulated sugar
Pinch of salt
½ cup water
1 cup hulled (green) pumpkin seeds, toasted

1. Preheat the oven to 375°F. Set a 2-quart soufflé dish or round ceramic casserole in the middle of the oven to preheat. Bring a pot of water to a boil.

2. In a dry, heavy, 2-quart saucepan, heat 1 cup of the granulated sugar over medium-low heat, stirring slowly with a fork, until the sugar melts and turns

golden brown. Cook, without stirring, swirling the pan, until the sugar is deep amber in color, about 5 minutes. This is your caramel. Remove the hot soufflé dish from the oven and immediately pour the caramel into the dish, tilting it to completely cover the bottom and sides. Set it aside to harden while you prepare the rest of the flan. (Leave the oven on.)

3. In a medium saucepan, combine the whole milk and the evaporated milk. Bring to a gentle simmer over medium heat, then remove from the heat. Pour the milk mixture through a fine-mesh sieve into a bowl; set aside.

4. In a large bowl using an electric mixer, beat together the remaining ¾ cup granulated sugar, the Hey Sugar!, and the eggs on medium speed until smooth and creamy. Beat in the salt, pumpkin, tequila, orange zest, cinnamon, ginger, cardamom, nutmeg, and vanilla. While stirring, add the strained milk mixture in a slow stream and stir until well combined.

5. Pour the custard over the caramel in the dish and set the dish in a roasting pan. Pour boiling water into the roasting pan until it comes about 1 inch up the sides of the soufflé dish. Put the pan in middle of the oven and reduce the oven temperature to 350°F. Bake until golden brown on top and a knife inserted into the center of the flan comes out clean, 1¼ to 1½ hours. Remove the dish from the water bath and transfer to a wire rack to cool. Refrigerate at least 6 hours.

6. Prepare the praline: Preheat the oven to 250°F. Line a baking sheet with aluminum foil and lightly oil the foil. Set the baking sheet in the oven to keep warm.

7. In a deep, heavy, 2-quart saucepan, combine the sugar, salt, and ½ cup water and cook over medium-low heat, stirring slowly with a fork, until

melted and pale golden. Cook the caramel without stirring, tilting the pan from side to side, until deep golden. Immediately stir in the pumpkin seeds and quickly pour the mixture onto the prepared baking sheet, spreading it into a thin sheet before it hardens. (If the caramel hardens and is difficult to spread, raise the oven temperature to 400°F and place the baking sheet in the oven until the caramel is warm enough to spread, 1 to 2 minutes.)

8. Let the praline cool on the baking sheet on a wire rack until completely hardened, then break it into large pieces.

9. To unmold the flan, run a thin knife around the edges to loosen it. Wiggle the dish from side to side; when the flan moves freely in the dish, invert a large serving platter with a lip over the dish. Holding the dish and platter securely together, quickly invert them together, turning the flan out onto the platter. The caramel will pool over and around it—this is exactly what you want to happen, so don't worry—it's normal. Cut the flan into wedges and serve with the caramel spooned over it, topped with shards of the praline.

CREATIVE BITES

CHOCOLATE-ALMOND DELIGHTS • *219*

BLACK SESAME–CACAO NIB BRITTLE • *222*

CARAMEL SUGAR HIGHS • *224*

FAREWELL TO PEACHES • *227*

GONE CRACKERS • *231*

AW, SNAP! MARGARITA BRITTLE • *233*

BAKED MERINGUE POMEGRANATE APPLES • *235*

SOME LIKE IT HOT MEXICAN-SPICED FUDGE • *239*

PEPPERMINT MARSHMALLOWS • *243*

POP STAR CARAMEL CORN • *246*

S'MORES • *249*

TRUE CONFECTIONS • *251*

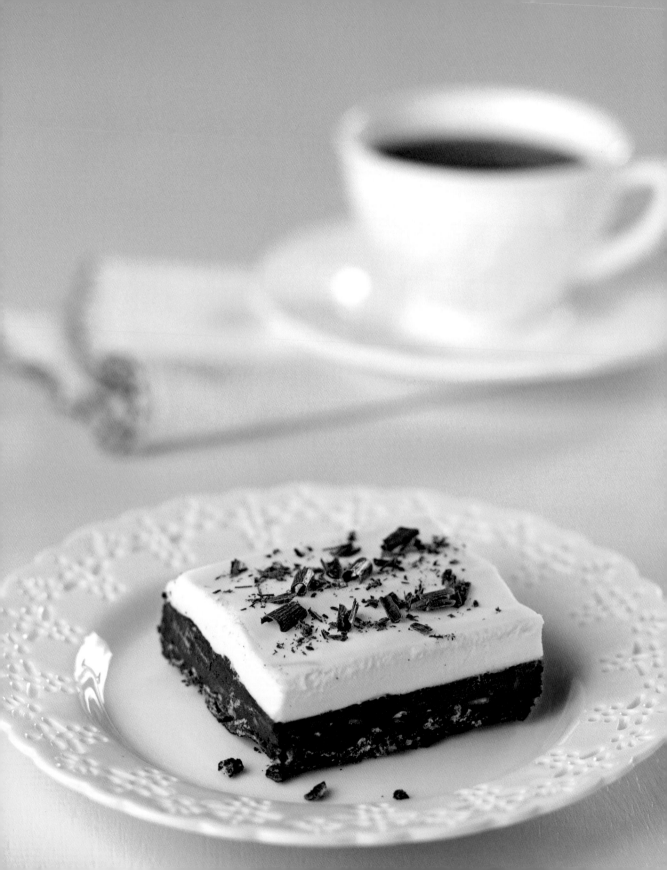

Chocolate-Almond Delights

This divine concoction (smooth meets crunchy!) is somewhere between a brownie and a pudding. Don't let the Frosted Flakes fool you—this is a high-brow sugar rush and tastes best on a fancy dessert plate, eaten with a fork.

Makes 9 bars

THC per serving: Please see page 54 to calculate.

Vegetable oil, for greasing the pan

Crust
4 ounces bittersweet chocolate
1 tablespoon Hey Sugar! (page 51)
3 cups Frosted Flakes cereal

Dark Chocolate–Almond Layer
8 ounces bittersweet chocolate
1 cup heavy cream
2 tablespoons Hey Sugar! (page 51)
2 tablespoons granulated sugar
2 tablespoons unsalted butter
½ cup raw almonds, toasted and coarsely chopped
1 tablespoon pure vanilla extract

White Chocolate Layer
2 teaspoons unflavored powdered gelatin
8 ounces white chocolate
1¾ cups heavy cream
1 teaspoon pure vanilla extract
¼ teaspoon almond extract
Chocolate shavings, for garnish

1. Grease a 9 x 13-inch baking pan with vegetable oil and line it with foil, pressing it into the corners and letting about 4 inches hang over two opposite sides of the pan. Grease the bottom and sides of the foil.

2. Prepare the crust: Set up a double boiler with 2 to 3 inches of water in the bottom pot and bring the water to a simmer. Melt the chocolate in the top section. Stir in the Hey Sugar! and Frosted Flakes. Pour the mixture into the prepared pan and spread it evenly. Refrigerate the crust while you prepare the dark chocolate layer.

3. Prepare the dark chocolate layer: Bring the water in the double boiler back to a simmer and place the chocolate in the top section. Melt the chocolate. Pour in the heavy cream, Hey Sugar!, and granulated sugar and stir until smooth and well combined. Add the butter, almonds, and vanilla and stir well to combine. Transfer the chocolate mixture to a bowl and set in the freezer until cool and thickened, 15 to 20 minutes. Stir well, then spread the dark chocolate layer evenly on top of the chilled crust. Refrigerate until firm, about 1 hour.

4. Prepare the white chocolate layer: Put ¼ cup water into a heat-proof measuring cup and sprinkle the gelatin over the water; let stand for 5 minutes. Meanwhile, fill a small saucepan halfway with water and heat over medium heat until just hot (not simmering). Reduce the heat to low, set the measuring cup in the saucepan, and stir until the gelatin has melted and the mixture is clear, 3 to 5 minutes. Remove from the heat.

5. Place the white chocolate in a bowl. In a small saucepan, heat ¾ cup of the heavy cream over medium heat until just simmering. Pour the cream over the white chocolate. Let stand until the chocolate has melted; stir until smooth. Using a rubber spatula, scrape in the warm gelatin mixture and

stir in the vanilla and almond extracts. Set in the freezer, stirring every few minutes, until cool.

6. In a medium bowl using an electric mixer, whip the remaining 1 cup heavy cream on medium-high speed until soft peaks form. Stir one-third of the whipped cream into the white chocolate mixture. Gently fold in the rest of the whipped cream. Spread the whipped cream evenly over the dark chocolate layer. Refrigerate until set, about 4 hours.

7. Run a knife around the edges of the pan to loosen the foil. Using the overhanging foil, lift the confection out of the pan and place it on a cutting board. Cut it into 9 equal-size squares, wiping the blade clean after each cut. Sprinkle chocolate shavings on top of each square.

8. Store in an airtight container in the refrigerator for up to 3 days.

Black Sesame-Cacao Nib Brittle

I dreamed up this creation after fans of our bakery raved about our margarita brittle. This delicious, unique brittle marries the rich, nutty flavor of toasted sesame seeds with the intense chocolaty flavor of cacao nibs.

Note: Keep a bowl of ice water close by, in case any of the hot sugar gets on your hands.

Makes 12 servings

THC per serving: Please see page 54 to calculate.

Vegetable oil, for greasing the pan
2 tablespoons salted butter
¾ cup granulated sugar
¼ cup Hey Sugar! (page 51)
⅛ teaspoon salt
½ cup raw almonds
1 tablespoon sesame seeds, toasted
2 teaspoons cacao nibs

1. Preheat the oven to 250°F. Grease an 8 x 8-inch baking pan with vegetable oil and line it with foil, pressing it into the corners and letting about 3 inches hang over two opposite sides of the pan. Grease the foil and place the pan in the warm oven until you are ready to use it.

2. In a medium saucepan, melt the butter over medium heat. Add the granulated sugar, Hey Sugar!, and salt and cook, stirring continuously, until the sugars have melted, 4 to 5 minutes, being careful not to let the sugar burn, which can happen quickly. (Remember to keep a bowl of ice water close by, in case any of the hot sugar gets on your hands.) The end color should be

dark amber. If it becomes grainy, reduce the heat and continue to stir, allowing the sugar to melt until smooth. Remove from the heat.

3. Add in the almonds, sesame seeds, and cacao nibs, and stir well. Pour the mixture into the warm pan and spread it evenly. Let cool completely.

4. Using the overhanging foil, lift the brittle out of the pan and place it on a flat surface. Invert, peel off the foil, and break into pieces. Place a large bowl on your scale and tare the scale. Place the brittle in the bowl and divide the weight by 12: This is your per-serving weight.

5. Store in an airtight container at room temperature for up to 2 weeks. Be sure to write the weight per serving on your storage container.

Caramel Sugar Highs

I top this delectable, sugary treat with a sprinkling of sea salt to create a crave-worthy combination of delightfulness. Cut into bite-size pieces and share!

Makes 48 squares

THC per serving: Please see page 54 to calculate.

Special equipment: candy thermometer or laser temperature gun (see note on high-altitude measurements on page 22)

Pastry

¼ cup Buddha Budda (page 43), slightly softened
¼ cup (4 tablespoons/½ stick) unsalted butter, slightly softened
1 cup powdered sugar
2 large eggs, beaten
2 cups all-purpose flour
1 teaspoon coarse salt
1 large egg white, lightly beaten

Caramel

¼ cup heavy cream
8 ounces bittersweet chocolate chips
2¼ cups granulated sugar
¼ cup Buddha Budda (page 43)
6 tablespoons unsalted butter
1 teaspoon pure vanilla extract
2½ teaspoons flaky sea salt, such as Maldon

1. Preheat the oven to 350°F. Line a 9 x 13-inch baking pan with aluminum foil, pressing it into the corners and leaving 2 inches hanging over on the short sides.

2. Prepare the pastry: In a large bowl using an electric mixer, cream together the Buddha Budda and butter on medium speed until well combined.

Reduce the mixer speed to low and add the powdered sugar. Add the eggs and beat until well combined. Add the flour and salt. Pour the mixture into the prepared pan, dampen your fingers, and press it into an even, ¼-inch-thick layer. Freeze until firm, at least 20 minutes.

3. Remove the pastry from the freezer and top it with a piece of parchment paper. Fill it with pie weights (if you don't have them, use uncooked rice or dried beans). Bake for 30 to 35 minutes, until just set. Carefully remove the pie weights and parchment paper. Brush the pastry shell with the egg white and bake for 10 to 15 minutes more, or until light golden brown. Let cool.

4. Prepare the caramel: In a medium saucepan, bring the cream to a simmer over medium heat, then reduce the heat to low and add the chocolate. Let stand for 1 minute, then stir until the chocolate has completely melted. Remove from the heat.

5. In a large, heavy saucepan, stir together the sugar and ¼ cup water. Bring to a simmer over medium heat, without stirring, and simmer until an amber-colored caramel forms, 7 to 10 minutes, then stir to blend in any crystals formed on the surface.

6. Remove the caramel from the heat and carefully stir in the chocolate-cream mixture. When the bubbling subsides, stir in the butter. Insert a candy thermometer or use your laser thermometer. Cook over medium-high heat, stirring with a wooden spoon, until the caramel reaches 240°F, 10 to 15 minutes. Let cool for 10 minutes, then stir in the vanilla and 1½ teaspoons of the salt. Pour the caramel over the cooled pastry. Refrigerate for 15 minutes.

7. Sprinkle the remaining 1 teaspoon salt on top of the caramel. Place back in the refrigerator and chill until firm, about 2 hours. Remove from the pan using the foil overhang and cut into 48 equal-size squares.

8. Store in an airtight container in the refrigerator for up to 2 weeks. Bring to room temperature before serving.

Farewell to Peaches

· ·

These grilled peach sundaes with Salted Caramel–Bourbon Sauce were originally created for a dinner party at the end of peach season, and they were quite a success. Decadent and delicious, you'll layer fresh peaches, sugared pecans, caramel, and tangy whipped cream, culminating in an explosion of flavor. But don't wait until the end of peach season: Make it as soon as fresh peaches are available.

Makes 4 servings

THC per serving: Please see page 54 to calculate.

Pecans
1 cup whole pecan halves
1½ tablespoons unsalted butter, melted
¾ teaspoon salt
¼ teaspoon cayenne pepper
1½ tablespoons Hey Sugar! (page 51)

Whipped Cream
1 cup heavy cream
3 tablespoons powdered sugar
1 teaspoon pure vanilla extract
¼ cup buttermilk

Peaches
4 ripe peaches
3 tablespoons olive oil
Salt

8 tablespoons Salted Caramel–Bourbon Sauce (page 274), for serving
Fresh rosemary, for garnish

1. Preheat the oven to 350°F.

2. Prepare the pecans: In a bowl, combine the pecans, melted butter, salt, and cayenne. Spread the pecans in a single layer on a nonstick baking sheet

and bake for 8 to 10 minutes, or until lightly toasted. Remove from the oven (leaving the oven on), sprinkle the Hey Sugar! over the nuts, and toss well. Bake for 2 to 3 minutes more. Remove from the oven and set aside to cool.

3. Prepare the whipped cream: In a medium bowl using an electric mixer, whip the cream on medium-high speed until soft peaks form. Reduce the mixer speed to low and add the powdered sugar and vanilla; once incorporated, raise the mixer speed to medium and whip until stiff peaks form. Slowly pour in the buttermilk and whip until well combined. Refrigerate until ready to use.

4. Prepare the peaches: Heat a charcoal grill to medium-low. Halve and pit the peaches (leave the skin on) and brush the cut sides with olive oil.

5. Place the peaches, cut side down, on the grill and cook until there are grill marks, about 2 minutes. Brush the peaches with oil again and sprinkle with salt. Flip onto the other side, brush with oil, and grill.

6. Place 2 peach halves in a bowl and top with a dollop of whipped cream. Sprinkle with pecans and drizzle each with 2 tablespoons of warm caramel sauce. Garnish with a tiny sprig of rosemary.

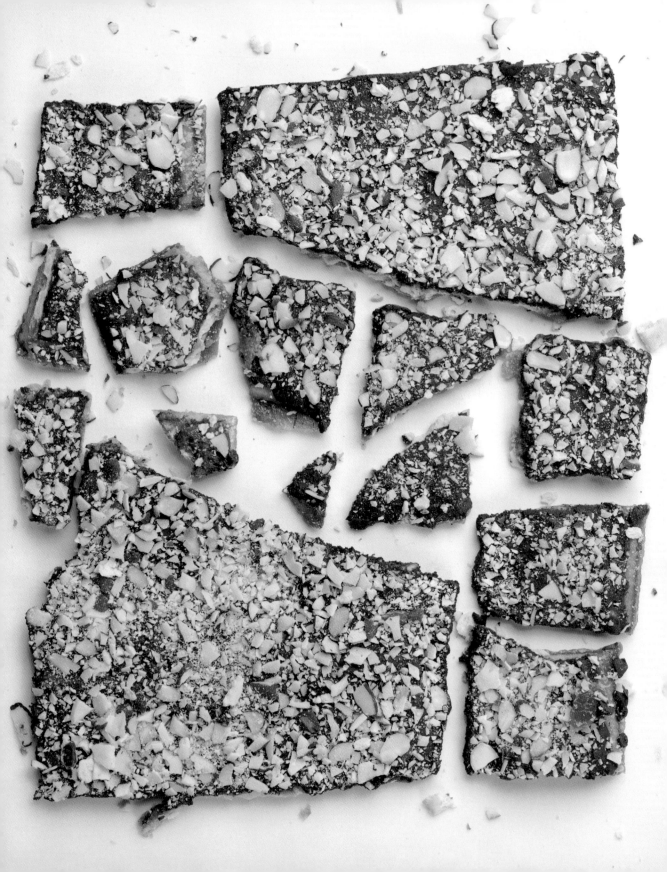

Gone Crackers

....

These will make you jump for joy when you take your first bite. Savor the amazing thing that happens when chocolate and toffee meet a salty base. With this recipe I wanted to create something that was easy enough for the most inexperienced baker while still being delicious enough for discerning palates. And you really can't go wrong with this flavor combination. After the first test run, I set this out for the staff to try after work. The entire tray went quickly—everyone went crazy for them. Which is where I got the name.

Makes 18 servings

THC per serving: Please see page 54 to calculate.

1½ sleeves saltine crackers (about 60 crackers)
¾ cup Buddha Budda (page 43)
¼ cup (4 tablespoons/½ stick) salted butter
1 cup packed dark brown sugar
8 ounces bittersweet chocolate, chopped
1 cup raw almonds, toasted and finely chopped

1. Preheat the oven to 400°F. Line a 10 x 15-inch jelly-roll pan with aluminum foil.

2. Arrange the crackers in a single layer on the prepared pan so that there are no empty spaces between them. Crush any crackers that do not fit on the pan into small crumbs and set aside.

3. In a medium saucepan, combine the Buddha Budda, butter, and sugar and bring to a rolling boil over medium heat. Remove from the heat and carefully pour the butter mixture over the crackers, covering them completely. Bake for 5 to 7 minutes, or until the toffee is bubbling. Remove from the oven and let cool for 1 minute.

4. Sprinkle the chopped chocolate on top of the hot toffee; allow to sit for 1 minute to soften and melt. With an offset spatula or a knife, spread the melted chocolate evenly over the toffee, then scatter the nuts and reserved crushed crackers over the top and gently press them into the chocolate layer. Refrigerate until firm and set, about 30 minutes.

5. Once set, break into small, uneven pieces. Place a large bowl on your scale and tare the scale. Place the toffee in the bowl and divide the weight by 18: This is your per-serving weight.

6. Store any uneaten toffee in an airtight container at room temperature for up to 2 weeks. Be sure to write the weight per serving on your storage container.

Aw, Snap! Margarita Brittle

....

I think of the sweet delicate toffee base of this brittle as an edible platform for the vibrant flavors of lime, pumpkin seeds, and tortilla chips. A splash of tequila brings it all together with a mischievous touch.

Makes 12 servings

THC per serving: Please see page 54 to calculate.

Vegetable shortening, for greasing the pan
2 tablespoons salted butter
¾ cup granulated sugar
¼ cup Hey Sugar! (page 51)
¼ teaspoon salt
½ cup hulled (green) pumpkin seeds, toasted
½ cup lightly crushed tortilla chips (about ¼-inch pieces)
2 tablespoons tequila
¼ teaspoon lime oil or extract

1. Preheat the oven to 250°F. Grease an 8 x 8-inch baking pan with vegetable shortening and line it with foil, pressing it into the corners and letting about 3 inches hang over two opposite sides of the pan. Grease the foil and place the baking pan in the warm oven until you are ready to use it.

2. In a medium saucepan, melt the butter over medium heat. Add the granulated sugar, Hey Sugar!, and salt and cook, stirring continuously, until the sugars are melted and the mixture is light amber in color, 4 to 5 minutes, being careful not to let the sugar burn, which can happen quickly. Remove from the heat.

3. Add in the pumpkin seeds, tortilla chips, tequila, and lime oil and stir well. Pour into the warm prepared pan and spread evenly. Let cool com-

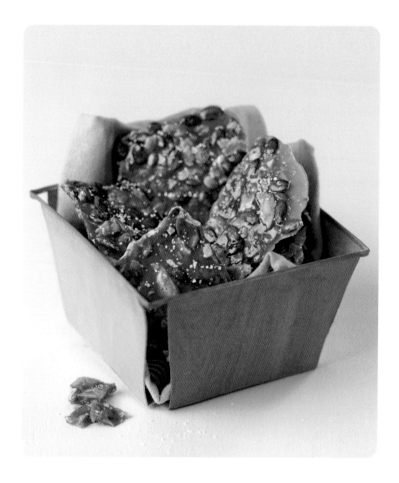

pletely. Using the overhanging foil, lift out of the pan and place on a flat surface.

4. Invert, peel off the foil, and snap into bite-size pieces. Place a large bowl on your scale and tare the scale. Place the brittle in the bowl and divide the weight by 12: This is your per-serving weight.

5. Store in an airtight container at room temperature for up to 2 weeks. Be sure to write the weight per serving on your storage container.

Baked Meringue Pomegranate Apples

Nothing *captures the cool-weather bounty of fall more eloquently than sweet, crisp apples, with their tantalizing fragrance and taste. One of my favorite things to do with apples is to bake them into a succulent dessert. I created this luscious meringue-coated baked fruit confection, filled with antioxidant-rich pomegranate seeds and walnuts, plus a dose of THC, to put a new spin on a quintessential treat. For the finishing touch, pour a lake of hot, caramel-y pomegranate syrup over each baked apple.*

Makes 6 baked apples

THC per serving: Please see page 54 to calculate.

Pomegranate Syrup
1 cup pure pomegranate juice
¼ cup honey
1 tablespoon pure vanilla extract

Baked Apples
6 medium baking apples, such as Honeycrisp or Cortland
½ cup fresh pomegranate seeds
¾ cup chopped walnuts
2 tablespoons Hey Sugar! (page 51)
6 tablespoons packed brown sugar
1 teaspoon lemon zest
6 cinnamon sticks

Meringue
6 egg whites
¼ teaspoon cream of tartar
½ cup granulated sugar
1 teaspoon pure vanilla extract

1. Preheat the oven to 350°F.

2. Prepare the pomegranate syrup: In a small saucepan, combine the pomegranate juice and honey and bring to a boil over medium heat. Reduce the heat to low and simmer, stirring occasionally, until the mixture has reduced by half. Let cool and stir in the vanilla. Set aside.

3. Prepare the apples: Wash the apples and remove the cores, but do not cut all the way through to the bottom. Peel off a wide strip (about 1½ inches) around the top edge. In a medium bowl, mix together the pomegranate seeds, walnuts, Hey Sugar!, brown sugar, and lemon zest. Divide the pomegranate mixture evenly among the apples, filling each apple to within ¼ inch of the top. Insert a cinnamon stick into the center of each apple.

4. Place the apples upright in a 9 x 13-inch baking dish. Pour the pomegranate syrup over the apples. Bake for 30 to 40 minutes, or until tender, basting frequently with the syrup in the pan.

5. While the apples are baking, prepare the meringue: In a medium bowl using an electric mixer, beat the egg whites with the cream of tartar on high speed until soft peaks form. Slowly add the granulated sugar and continue beating until stiff and shiny. Blend in the vanilla extract.

6. Remove the apples from the oven and raise the oven temperature to 450°F. Spoon or pipe meringue in decorative swirls over the upper one-third of each apple. Return the apples to the oven and bake for 3 to 4 minutes more, or until the meringue is golden brown. Watch carefully to avoid burning.

7. To serve, evenly distribute the hot pomegranate syrup from the baking dish among six plates and place a baked apple on top. Remove the cinnamon stick before eating.

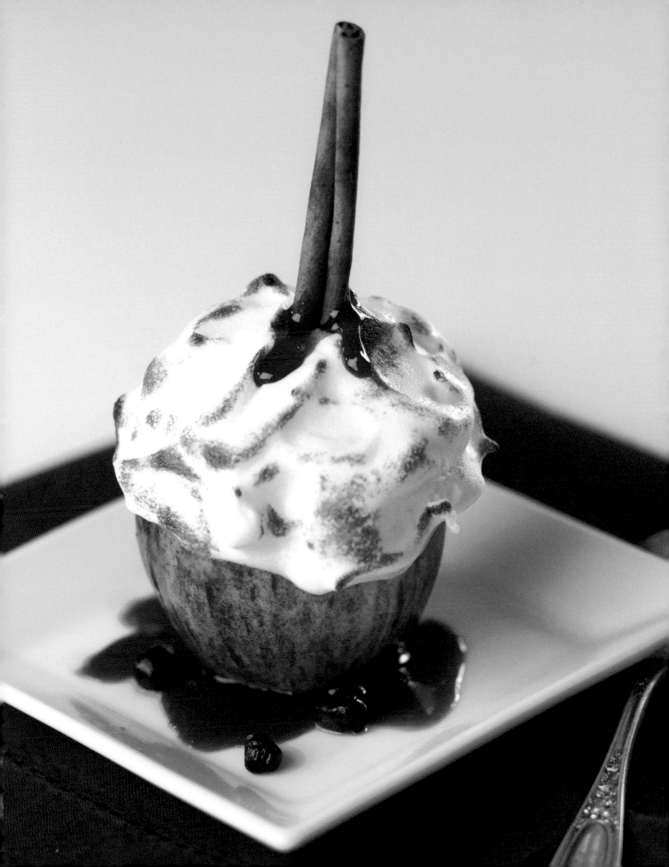

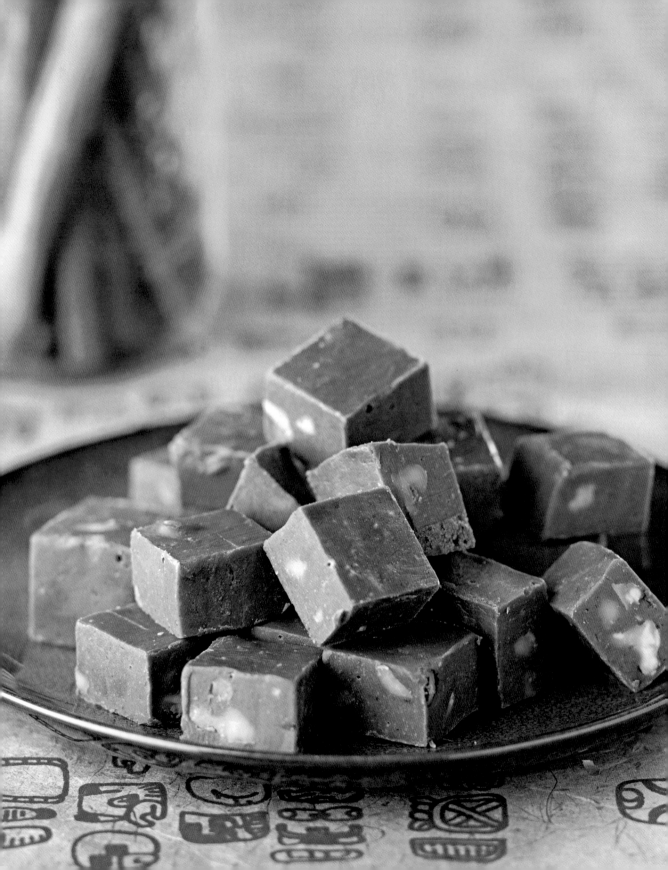

Some Like It Hot Mexican-Spiced Fudge

This chocolate-butterscotch fudge spiced with chile will appeal to anyone who likes a little heat with her sugar. Grace Gutierrez, head baker at Sweet Mary Jane, developed the recipe when we wanted to spice up the menu. It was a hit from the get-go. Heat, stir, blend, chill, and let the fiesta begin.

Makes 81 pieces

THC per serving: Please see page 54 to calculate.

Vegetable shortening, for greasing the pan
1 (14-ounce) can sweetened condensed milk
¼ cup Hey Sugar! (page 51)
1 (12-ounce) bag milk chocolate chips
1 (12-ounce) bag butterscotch chips
2 tablespoons unsalted butter
2 teaspoons pure vanilla extract
1 teaspoon ground cinnamon
½ teaspoon cayenne pepper
½ teaspoon ancho chile powder
¾ cup chopped walnuts (optional)

1. Grease a 9 x 9-inch pan with vegetable shortening.

2. Bring about 1 inch of water to a simmer in a medium saucepan. Set a medium heat-proof bowl over the simmering water, being sure the bottom of the bowl does not touch the water. Place the condensed milk, Hey Sugar!, milk chocolate chips, butterscotch chips, and butter in the bowl and heat until the chips are melted and the mixture is smooth and creamy.

3. Remove from the heat. Add the vanilla, cinnamon, cayenne, ancho chile powder, and walnuts (if using) to the warm chocolate mixture and stir to combine.

4. Pour the mixture into the prepared pan. Refrigerate until set, 1 to 1½ hours. Cut into 81 equal-size squares.

5. Store in an airtight container lined with waxed paper. Separate each layer of fudge with additional layers of waxed paper. Store in the refrigerator for up to 6 weeks, or in the freezer for up to 6 months.

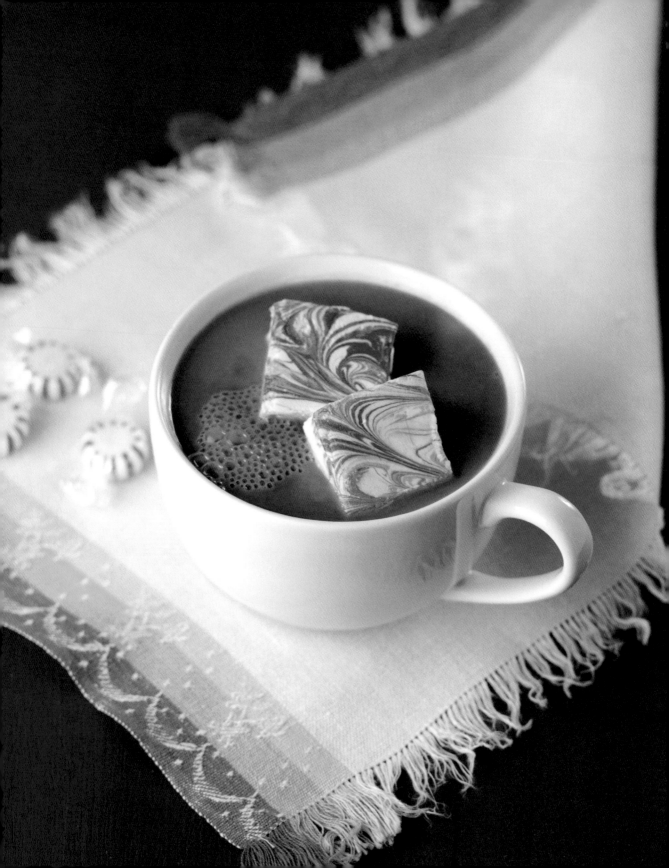

Peppermint Marshmallows

I came up with the idea of making infused marshmallows when a group of back-packers were looking for something to take with them on a weeklong journey into the Rockies. They wanted a confection that would last in the heat, in a backpack. The marshmallows were a huge success, a perfect way to make s'mores extra special. The idea of adding peppermint came later that year, when fans of Sweet Mary Jane asked for a seasonal treat to give as a holiday gift. Drop into your favorite cup of hot cocoa (or just eat them as they are!), sit by the fire, and enjoy.

Makes 36 marshmallows

THC per serving: Please see page 54 to calculate.

Special equipment: candy thermometer or laser temperature gun
    (see note on high-altitude measurements on page 22)
Nonstick vegetable oil spray, for greasing the pan
½ cup powdered sugar
1½ cups plus 2 tablespoons granulated sugar
6 tablespoons Hey Sugar! (page 51)
½ cup light corn syrup
4 (¼-ounce) packages unflavored powdered gelatin
1 teaspoon peppermint extract (optional; see Note, page 245)
2 large egg whites
2 teaspoons red food coloring (optional; see Note, page 245)
Candy canes (optional)

1. Coat a 13 x 9-inch rectangular metal baking pan (if you want thicker marshmallows, use a 9 x 9-inch pan) with nonstick cooking spray and dust the bottom and sides with powdered sugar. Reserve any remaining sugar for later use.

2. In a small saucepan, combine the granulated sugar, Hey Sugar!, corn syrup, and ¾ cup water; heat over medium heat, stirring, until the sugar has

dissolved. Stop stirring and let the mixture come to a boil. Raise the heat to medium-high and cook until the mixture registers 260°F on a candy thermometer. Remove from the heat.

3. Put ¾ cup water into a heat-proof glass bowl and sprinkle the gelatin over the water; let stand for 5 minutes. Meanwhile, fill a small saucepan halfway with water and heat over medium heat until just hot (not simmering). Reduce the heat to low, set the bowl over the saucepan, and stir until the gelatin has melted and the mixture is clear, 3 to 5 minutes. Remove from the heat. Stir in the peppermint extract (if using). Set aside.

4. In a large bowl using an electric mixer, or in the bowl of a stand mixer fitted with the wire whisk, beat the egg whites until stiff (but not dry) peaks form. Combine the gelatin and the sugar syrup. With the mixer running, gradually add the gelatin-sugar mixture to the egg whites. Mix on high speed until very thick and tripled in volume, 12 to 15 minutes.

5. Pour the mixture into the prepared pan. Working quickly, drop dots of food coloring across the surface of the marshmallow (if using food coloring). With a toothpick, swirl the food coloring into the marshmallow to create a marbled effect. If you want to get fancy, crush up candy canes and sprinkle them over the top, then lightly press them into the marshmallow.

6. Let the marshmallow stand, uncovered, at room temperature until firm, at least 3 hours, or overnight. Run a thin knife around the edges of the pan and invert the pan onto a large cutting board. Lift up one corner of the inverted pan and carefully loosen the marshmallow so it falls onto the cut-

ting board. Cut the marshmallow into 36 equal-size squares. Dust with the remaining powdered sugar.

7. Store in an airtight container at room temperature for up to 1 week.

Note: *When making these for the S'Mores recipe on page 249, substitute vanilla extract for the peppermint and leave out the food coloring.*

Pop Star Caramel Corn

This sweet-salty, melty-crunchy, on-the-go treat sells like crazy at Sweet Mary Jane. Have all your ingredients measured out and ready to go, as the recipe comes together quickly. A kernel of wisdom: Be sure to stick to the proper doses, as this is one of those things that you just can't stop eating.

Makes 18 servings (about ½ cup per serving)

THC per serving: Please see page 54 to calculate.

9 cups popped popcorn (⅓ cup kernels prepared any way you like, or microwave popcorn)
1 cup cashews (optional)
¾ cup Buddha Budda (page 43)
¼ cup (4 tablespoons/½ stick) salted butter
2 cups firmly packed light brown sugar
½ cup light corn syrup
1 teaspoon salt
¾ teaspoon baking soda
2 teaspoons pure vanilla extract

1. Preheat the oven to 250°F.

2. Place the popcorn and the cashews (if using) into a very large bowl. You are going to be pouring the caramel over the popcorn, so give yourself room to mix everything.

3. In a large saucepan, melt the Buddha Budda and butter over medium heat. Stir in the brown sugar, corn syrup, and salt. Stirring continuously, bring to a gentle boil. Stop stirring and allow to boil for 4 minutes (2 minutes at high altitude).

4. Remove from the heat and stir in the baking soda and vanilla; mix well.

Pour the caramel over the popcorn; use a rubber spatula to gently fold the caramel into the popcorn mixture until all the popcorn is coated evenly. Spread the popcorn mixture on two large baking sheets. Bake for 1 hour, stirring every 15 minutes. Remove from the oven and let cool.

5. When cool enough to handle, break into pieces. Place a large bowl on your scale and tare the scale. Pour in the Pop Star and divide the weight by 18: This is the per-serving weight.

6. Store in an airtight container at room temperature for up to 2 months. Be sure to write the weight per serving on your storage container.

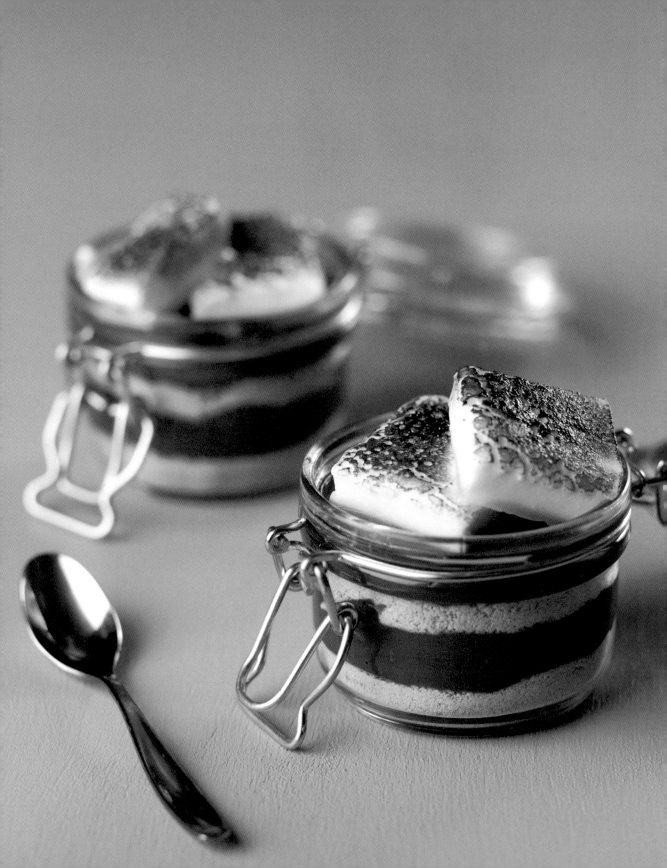

S'mores

This tiny, ever-so-sweet treat is easy and fun, and the scent of toasted marshmallows filling the room is like having a little camping trip in your kitchen.

Makes 2 servings

THC per serving: Please see page 54 to calculate.

Special equipment: two 4-ounce heat-proof jars, such as mason jars; butane torch

½ cup graham cracker crumbs (from about 5 or 6 graham crackers)

½ cup Nutella

4 Marshmallows (page 243)

1. In each mason jar, place one-quarter of the graham cracker crumbs and then one-quarter of the Nutella. Repeat once more. Top each with 2 marshmallows.

2. Using a butane torch, carefully toast the marshmallows until they are just lightly golden brown and melty. (If you don't have a torch, you can pop them under the broiler.) Serve.

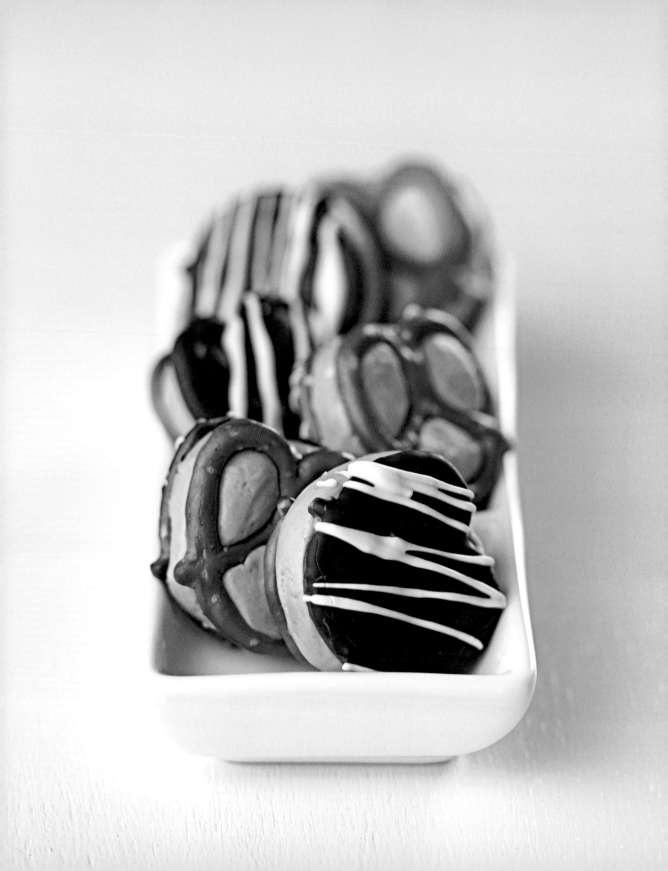

True Confections

This recipe hits the sweet-salty nail on the head, with a bite-size peanut butter–and-pretzel confection all wrapped up in a cloak of semisweet chocolate. A Sweet Mary Jane classic.

Makes 24 pretzel sandwiches

THC per serving: Please see page 54 to calculate.

Filling
¾ cup creamy peanut butter
¼ cup Buddha Budda (page 43), slightly softened
2 teaspoons pure vanilla extract
2 to 2½ cups powdered sugar
48 pretzels (we used Rold Gold mini low-fat pretzels)

Glaze
6 ounces semisweet chocolate chips
2 teaspoons vegetable shortening

Drizzle
¼ cup white chocolate chips
¼ teaspoon vegetable shortening

1. Weigh the bowl that you will be using to hold the finished dough and write down this number. Line a baking sheet with parchment paper.

2. In the bowl you weighed previously, using an electric mixer, beat together the peanut butter, Buddha Budda, and vanilla on medium speed until well blended.

3. Reduce the mixer speed to low and gradually add 2 cups of the powdered sugar. You want the dough to be soft enough to shape but not sticky. Add more sugar if the dough is too sticky to handle.

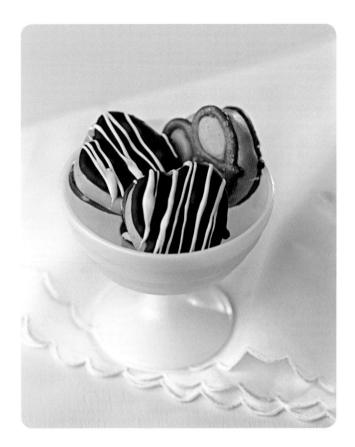

4. Weigh the dough, subtract the weight of the bowl, and divide by 24: This is your filling-per–pretzel sandwich weight. Place a small piece of parchment paper on your scale. Weigh out the dough for each pretzel sandwich and roll into a smooth ball. Place the dough ball on top of one pretzel, top with second pretzel, and gently press together, being careful not to break the pretzels. (The filling and the pretzels must stay together; otherwise, when you dip them in the chocolate, they will fall apart.) Place the pretzel sandwiches on the prepared baking sheet. Refrigerate for 30 minutes.

5. Prepare the glaze: Set up a double boiler with 2 to 3 inches of water in the bottom and bring the water to a simmer. Place the semisweet chocolate and shortening in the top section and stir continuously until the chocolate has melted, being careful not to get any water in the chocolate or it will seize. When the chocolate is completely melted, remove it from the heat.

6. Pick up a pretzel sandwich and dip only one side into the chocolate. Return the dipped pretzel to the baking sheet with the undipped side down. Continue until all the pretzel sandwiches have been dipped. Refrigerate until the glaze has set.

7. Prepare the drizzle: Return the water in the double boiler to a simmer and place the white chocolate and shortening in the top section. Stir continuously until the chocolate has melted, being careful not to get any water in the chocolate or it will seize. Place the pretzel sandwiches dipped side down on a wire rack set over a sheet of waxed paper. Dip a fork into the melted chocolate and drizzle it over the pretzel sandwiches.

8. Store in an airtight container in the refrigerator for up to 10 days.

TRUFFLES

ALOHA TRUFFLES · *257*

CHAI HIGH TRUFFLES · *259*

KEY LIME KICKERS · *261*

LATE-NIGHT SNACK TRUFFLES · *263*

MALTED MILK TRUFFLES · *265*

420 抹茶 MATCHA-SAMA TRUFFLES · *267*

SCOUT'S HONOR · *269*

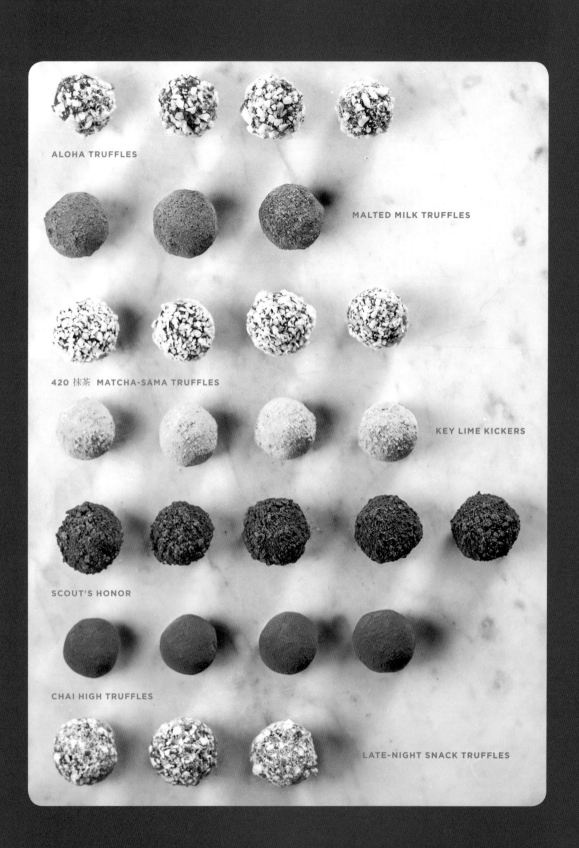

ALOHA TRUFFLES

MALTED MILK TRUFFLES

420 抹茶 MATCHA-SAMA TRUFFLES

KEY LIME KICKERS

SCOUT'S HONOR

CHAI HIGH TRUFFLES

LATE-NIGHT SNACK TRUFFLES

Aloha Truffles

These sophisticated truffles meld the magic of chocolate with the tropical tastes of coconut and macadamia nuts.

⌐꒐ *Makes 24 truffles*

THC per serving: Please see page 54 to calculate.

6 tablespoons heavy cream
1 teaspoon pure coconut extract (see Note, page 258)
2 tablespoons unsalted butter
1 teaspoon corn syrup
¼ cup Hey Sugar! (page 51)
10 ounces good-quality dark chocolate, coarsely chopped
Unsweetened shredded coconut and finely chopped macadamia nuts,
    for rolling

1. Weigh the bowl that will hold the finished ganache and write down this number. Set up a double boiler with 2 to 3 inches of water in the bottom pot and bring the water to a simmer. Pour the cream in the top section and heat until it begins to simmer gently.

2. Reduce the heat to low. Stir in the butter, corn syrup, and Hey Sugar!. When well combined, add the chocolate and stir well. When the ganache is smooth, remove from the heat and stir in the coconut extract. Wipe the water off the bottom and sides of the pan (you don't want any water dripping into the ganache) and pour the ganache into the bowl you weighed previously. Place in the freezer for 45 to 60 minutes, or until the ganache is firm but pliable. If the mixture becomes too solid, let it sit at room temperature until it softens.

3. Place the shredded coconut in one bowl and the macadamia nuts in another. Line two baking sheets with parchment paper. Weigh the ganache, subtract the weight of the bowl, and divide by 24: This is your per-truffle weight. Using a spoon, scoop out the ganache, weigh to make sure it's the correct portion, and set on one of the prepared baking sheets. Using your hands, quickly roll the ganache into balls and then roll them in either the coconut or macadamia nuts to coat completely.

4. Set the coated truffle on the second prepared baking sheet. Cover and store in the refrigerator for up to 5 weeks. The truffles are best served at room temperature.

Note: You can find coconut extract in most good supermarkets or natural food stores.

Chai High Truffles

White chocolate and chai come together to make this little cloud of a truffle. Watch as they disappear before your very eyes.

_____ 🖎 *Makes 24 truffles*

THC per serving: Please see page 54 to calculate.

7 tablespoons heavy cream
3 chai tea bags
1 teaspoon corn syrup
¼ cup Hey Sugar! (page 51)
2 tablespoons unsalted butter
10 ounces white chocolate, coarsely chopped
¼ cup unsweetened cocoa powder

1. Weigh the bowl that will hold the finished ganache and write down this number. Set up a double boiler with 2 to 3 inches of water in the bottom pot and bring the water to a simmer. Pour the cream in the top section and heat until it begins to simmer gently. Remove the top section from the heat. Place the tea bags in the cream and let steep for 5 minutes. Remove the tea bags, gently pressing out as much liquid as you can without breaking the bag. (Don't worry if a few tea leaves get into the cream.)

2. Return the top section with the infused cream onto the bottom of the double boiler. Reduce the heat to low. Stir in the corn syrup, Hey Sugar!, and butter. When well combined, add the white chocolate and stir well. When the ganache is smooth, remove from the heat. Wipe the water off the bottom and sides of the pan (you don't want any water dripping into the ganache) and pour the ganache into the bowl you weighed previously. Let cool, then place in the freezer for 45 to 60 minutes, or until the ganache is firm but pliable.

3. Place the cocoa powder in a shallow bowl. Line two baking sheets with parchment paper. Weigh the ganache, subtract the weight of the bowl, and divide by 24: This is your per-truffle weight. Using a spoon, scoop out the ganache, weigh to make sure it's the correct portion, and set on one of the prepared baking sheets. Using your hands, quickly roll the ganache into balls and then roll them in the cocoa powder to coat completely.

4. Set the truffles on the second prepared baking sheet. Cover and store in the refrigerator for up to 5 weeks. The truffles are best served at room temperature.

Key Lime Kickers

These truffles are like tiny key lime pies, and we can't make them fast enough at Sweet Mary Jane. A patient favorite, they won first place in two categories (Best Edibles and Patients' Choice) at the 2013 Hemp Connoisseur/THC Classic. Key lime oil can be found in craft shops and natural food grocers, or ordered online.

Makes 24 truffles

THC per serving: Please see page 54 to calculate.

6 tablespoons heavy cream
2 tablespoons unsalted butter
1 teaspoon light corn syrup
¼ cup Hey Sugar! (page 51)
10 ounces good-quality white chocolate, coarsely chopped
8 drops pure key lime oil
Graham cracker crumbs, for coating

1. Weigh the bowl that will hold the finished ganache and write down this number. Set up a double boiler with 2 to 3 inches of water in the bottom pot and bring the water to a simmer. Pour the cream in the top section and heat until it begins to simmer gently.

2. Stir in the butter, corn syrup, and Hey Sugar!. When well combined, add the white chocolate; stir well. When the ganache is smooth, remove the top section of the double boiler from the heat and add the key lime oil, stirring to combine. Wipe the water off the bottom and sides of the pan (you don't want any water dripping into the ganache) and pour the ganache into the bowl you weighed previously. Place in the freezer for 45 to 60 minutes, or until the ganache is firm but pliable.

3. Place the graham cracker crumbs in a shallow bowl. Line two baking sheets with parchment paper. Weigh the ganache, subtract the weight of the bowl, and divide by 24: This is your per-truffle weight. Using a spoon, scoop out the ganache, weigh to make sure it's the correct portion, and set on one of the prepared baking sheets. Using your hands, quickly roll the ganache into balls and then roll in the graham cracker crumbs to coat completely.

4. Set the truffles on the second prepared baking sheet. Cover and store in the refrigerator for up to 5 weeks. The truffles are best served at room temperature.

Late-Night Snack Truffles

··

So, you can't sleep? One of these might do the trick. The ingredients in this truffle work so well together—sweet, silky chocolate and salty chips rolled in pretzel crumbs for crunch. Take a bite—mmm, sooo good. Sigh. Now go to bed.

Makes 24 truffles

THC per serving: Please see page 54 to calculate.

6 tablespoons heavy cream
2 tablespoons unsalted butter
1 teaspoon light corn syrup
¼ cup Hey Sugar! (page 51)
10 ounces good-quality dark chocolate, coarsely chopped
1 teaspoon pure vanilla extract
½ cup finely crushed potato chips
Finely crushed pretzel crumbs, for coating

1. Weigh the bowl that will hold the finished ganache and write down this number. Set up a double boiler with 2 to 3 inches of water in the bottom pot and bring the water to a simmer. Pour the cream into the top section, and heat until it begins to simmer gently.

2. Stir in the butter, corn syrup, and Hey Sugar!. When well combined, add the chocolate. Stir well. When the ganache is smooth, remove from the heat and add the vanilla and potato chips, stirring to combine. Wipe the water off the bottom and sides of the pan (you don't want any water dripping into the ganache) and pour the ganache into the bowl you weighed previously. Place in the freezer for 45 to 60 minutes, or until the ganache is firm but pliable.

3. Place the pretzel crumbs in a shallow bowl. Line two baking sheets with parchment paper. Weigh the ganache, subtract the weight of the bowl, and

divide by 24: This is your per-truffle weight. Using a spoon, scoop out the ganache, weigh to make sure it's the correct portion, and set on one of the prepared baking sheets. Using your hands, quickly roll the ganache into balls and then roll in the crushed pretzel crumbs to coat completely.

4. Set the truffles on the second prepared baking sheet. Cover and store in the refrigerator for up to 5 weeks. The truffles are best served at room temperature.

Malted Milk Truffles

❋ ···

My childlike excitement for this drugstore candy (i.e., the giant box of malted milk balls) has taken a backseat to a love of more worldly confections, like these easy-to-prepare delights.

Makes 24 truffles

THC per serving: Please see page 54 to calculate.

6 tablespoons heavy cream
2 tablespoons unsalted butter
1 teaspoon light corn syrup
¼ cup Hey Sugar! (page 51)
8 tablespoons malted milk powder
15 ounces good-quality milk chocolate, coarsely chopped
1 tablespoon unsweetened cocoa powder
5 tablespoons plus 4 tablespoons malted milk powder

1. Weigh the bowl that will hold the finished ganache and write down this number. Set up a double boiler with 2 to 3 inches of water in the bottom pot and bring the water to a simmer. Pour the cream in the top section, and heat until it begins to simmer gently.

2. Stir in the butter, corn syrup, Hey Sugar!, and 5 tablespoons of the malted milk powder. When well combined, add the chocolate. Stir well. When the ganache is smooth, remove the top double boiler section from the heat. Wipe the water off the bottom and sides of the pan (you don't want any water dripping into the ganache) and pour the ganache into the bowl you weighed previously. Place in the freezer for 45 to 60 minutes, or until the ganache is firm but pliable. If the mixture becomes too solid, let it sit at room temperature until it softens.

3. In a shallow bowl, mix the cocoa powder and the remaining 3 tablespoons malted milk powder together. Line two baking sheets with parchment paper. Weigh the ganache, subtract the weight of the bowl, and divide by 24: This is your per-truffle weight. Using a spoon, scoop out the ganache, weigh to make sure it's the correct portion, and set on one of the prepared baking sheets. Using your hands, quickly roll the ganache into balls and then roll them in the malted milk powder mixture to coat completely.

4. Set the truffles on the second prepared baking sheet. Cover and store in the refrigerator for up to 5 weeks. The truffles are best served at room temperature.

420 抹茶 Matcha-Sama Truffles

I love the balance of components here: dark chocolate, pleasantly bitter matcha green tea flavor, and unsweetened coconut. Sweet surrender.

This truffle made its debut on April 20, an important date and a big holiday in Colorado, "420" (4/20) being a symbol for marijuana culture. There are a number of stories about where this term came from. In the most popular tale, the use of 420 started in San Rafael, California, in the early 1970s. It was deemed the "hour of cannabis consumption" (much like an older generation's cocktail hour!) by a group of high school students known as "The Waldos." You can read more about 420 on my website.

Makes 24 truffles

THC per serving: Please see page 54 to calculate.

6 tablespoons heavy cream
2 tablespoons unsalted butter
1 teaspoon light corn syrup
¼ cup Hey Sugar! (page 51)
1 teaspoon matcha green tea powder
10 ounces good-quality dark chocolate, coarsely chopped
¼ cup shredded unsweetened coconut
¼ cup unsweetened cocoa powder

1. Weigh the bowl that will hold the finished ganache and write down this number. Set up a double boiler with 2 to 3 inches of water in the bottom pot. Pour the cream in the top section and heat until it begins to simmer gently.

2. Stir in the butter, corn syrup, Hey Sugar!, and matcha. When well combined, add the chocolate. Stir well. When the ganache is smooth, remove the top double boiler section from the heat. Wipe the water off the bottom and sides of the pan (you don't want any water dripping into the ganache) and

pour the ganache into the bowl you weighed previously. Place in the freezer for 45 to 60 minutes, or until the ganache is firm but pliable.

3. Place the shredded coconut and the cocoa powder in separate shallow bowls. Line two baking sheets with parchment paper. Weigh the ganache, subtract the weight of the bowl, and divide by 24: This is your per-truffle weight. Using a spoon, scoop out the ganache, weigh to make sure it's the correct portion, and set on one of the prepared baking sheets. Using your hands, quickly roll the ganache into balls and then roll them in either the shredded coconut or the cocoa powder to coat completely.

4. Set the truffles on the second prepared baking sheet. Cover and store in the refrigerator for up to 5 weeks. The truffles are best served at room temperature.

Scout's Honor

I wanted a great addition to the Sweet Mary Jane menu and came up with this recipe after reading a story in the newspaper about an enterprising young Girl Scout who sold cookies in front of a dispensary—and made a killing doing it! Well, who doesn't love Thin Mint Girl Scout cookies? Almost instantly, these became one of our top sellers.

Makes 24 truffles

THC per serving: Please see page 54 to calculate.

6 tablespoons heavy cream
2 tablespoons unsalted butter
1 teaspoon light corn syrup
¼ cup Hey Sugar! (page 51)
10 ounces good-quality dark chocolate, coarsely chopped
1 teaspoon mint extract
1 (9-ounce) package Thin Mint Girl Scout cookies,
    or ½ package Keebler Grasshopper cookies, finely ground in food processor

1. Weigh the bowl that will hold the finished ganache and write down this number. Set up a double boiler with 2 to 3 inches of water in the bottom pot and bring the water to a simmer. Pour the cream into the top section and heat until it begins to simmer gently.

2. Stir in the butter, corn syrup, and Hey Sugar!. When well combined, add the chocolate. Stir well. When the ganache is smooth, remove the top section of the double boiler from the heat and add the mint extract, stirring to combine. Wipe the water off the bottom and sides of the pan (you don't want any water dripping into the ganache) and pour the ganache into the bowl you weighed previously. Place in the freezer for 45 to 60 minutes, or until the ganache is firm but pliable.

3. Place the cookie crumbs in a shallow bowl. Line two baking sheets with parchment paper. Weigh the ganache, subtract the weight of the bowl, and divide by 24: This is your per-truffle weight. Using a spoon, scoop out the ganache, weigh to make sure it's the correct portion, and set on one of the prepared baking sheets. Using your hands, quickly roll the ganache into balls and then roll them in the cookie crumbs to coat completely.

4. Set the truffles on the second prepared baking sheet. Cover and store in the refrigerator for up to 5 weeks. The truffles are best served at room temperature. Store any leftover cookie crumbs in an airtight container.

SAUCES

ECSTASY SAUCE · *273*

SALTED CARAMEL-BOURBON SAUCE · *274*

SILKY SWEET PEANUT BUTTER SAUCE · *275*

MAGIC MOMENT SAUCE · *276*

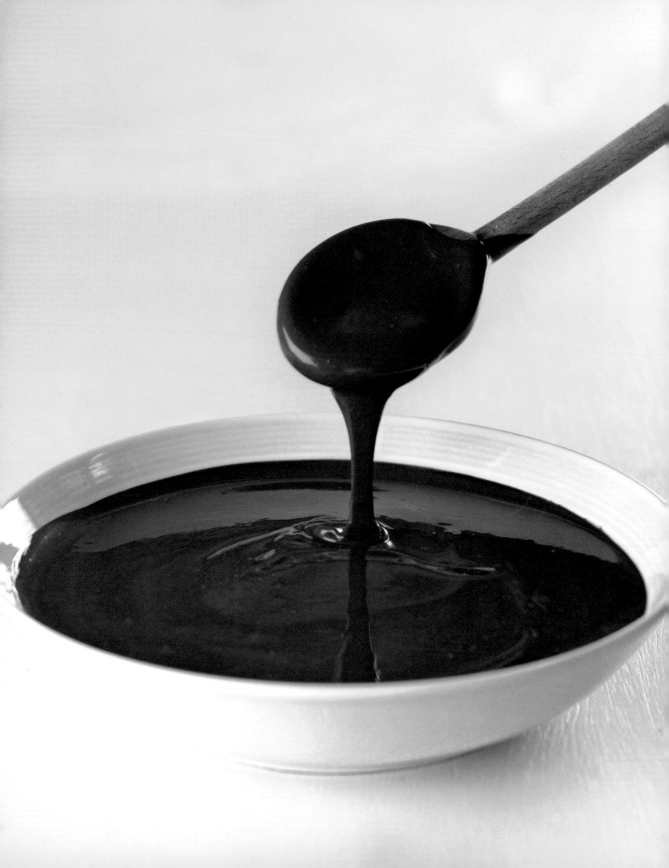

Ecstasy Sauce

This honey-kissed, creamy, chocolatey sauce is perfect for dipping farm-fresh fruit. Or drizzle it over your favorite ice cream. Or put some pieces of cubed angel food or pound cake on a toothpick and treat it like fondue. Does all that seem like too much? Then just take a spoonful fresh from the fridge. Aren't you saucy!

Makes 1½ to 2 cups sauce

THC per serving: Please see page 54 to calculate.

¾ cup granulated sugar
3 tablespoons Hey Sugar! (page 51)
½ cup unsweetened cocoa powder
⅔ cup evaporated milk
⅓ cup honey
⅓ cup salted butter
1 tablespoon pure vanilla extract

1. In a medium saucepan, combine the granulated sugar, Hey Sugar!, cocoa powder, evaporated milk, and honey and cook over medium heat, stirring continuously, until the mixture begins to boil. Without stirring, simmer for 5 to 7 minutes, until the mixture comes to a slow boil. Remove from the heat and stir in the butter and vanilla.

2. Let the sauce cool slightly, then pour into a glass jar and refrigerate. The sauce will keep in the refrigerator for up to 1 month. Reheat before using.

Salted Caramel–Bourbon Sauce

Try this over your favorite ice cream, frozen yogurt, pancakes, or Farewell to Peaches (page 227).

Makes 1 cup sauce

THC per serving: Please see page 54 to calculate.

½ cup granulated sugar
2 tablespoons plus 2 teaspoons Hey Sugar! (page 51)
3 tablespoons bourbon
¼ cup heavy cream
3 tablespoons unsalted butter, cut into 6 cubes, slightly softened
½ teaspoon coarse salt
1 teaspoon pure vanilla extract

1. In a small pot, heat the granulated sugar, Hey Sugar!, and 2 tablespoons of the bourbon over medium-low heat, stirring continuously, until the sugar has dissolved and the mixture is smooth. Raise the heat to medium and let the mixture come to a boil without stirring. Boil (a gentle, not rolling, boil) for 6 to 8 minutes (at high altitude, boil for 3 to 4 minutes), swirling the pot every 30 seconds and wiping down the sides of the pot with a wet pastry brush to prevent sugar from sticking to the sides and crystallizing.

2. When the mixture is thick and deep golden, remove from the heat. Slowly pour in the heavy cream, whisking continuously (the mixture will bubble). Stir in the butter and salt. When the mixture is well blended, remove from the heat and let cool for 5 minutes. Stir in the vanilla and the remaining 1 tablespoon bourbon.

3. Let the caramel cool slightly, then pour into a glass jar and refrigerate. The sauce will keep in the refrigerator for up to 1 month.

Silky Sweet Peanut Butter Sauce

Smooth and luscious. Decadent and dreamy. Serve piping hot over ice cream (of course), pancakes, or waffles, or in a Sweet Mary Jane favorite: Pop Star Peanut Butter Parfait (page 205).

Makes about 2 cups sauce

THC per serving: Please see page 54 to calculate.

½ cup plus 3 tablespoons firmly packed light brown sugar
5 tablespoons Hey Sugar! (page 51)
½ cup light corn syrup
¼ cup (4 tablespoons/½ stick) unsalted butter
½ teaspoon salt
1 cup creamy peanut butter
½ cup evaporated milk
1 tablespoon pure vanilla extract
1 teaspoon ground cinnamon

1. In a small saucepan, combine the brown sugar, Hey Sugar!, corn syrup, butter, and salt and bring to a boil over medium heat, stirring occasionally. Reduce the heat to low and add the peanut butter, stirring until the mixture is smooth. Add the evaporated milk and stir well. Stir in the vanilla and cinnamon. Remove from the heat. Serve warm.

2. Let any remaining peanut butter sauce cool, then pour into a glass jar and refrigerate. The sauce will keep in the refrigerator for up to 2 months. Reheat before using.

Magic Moment Sauce

....

Remember when you were a kid and you'd order soft-serve ice cream dipped in chocolate? The chocolate sauce would instantly, miraculously form a delicious, hard shell around the outside of the cold ice cream. Now, you can pour this sauce over your favorite ice cream, sit back, and watch the magic again.

Makes ¾ cup sauce

THC per serving: Please see page 54 to calculate.

¼ cup Coconut Bliss (page 46)
¼ cup coconut oil
16 ounces good-quality semisweet or bittersweet chocolate, chopped
1 tablespoon pure vanilla extract
½ teaspoon instant espresso powder
¼ teaspoon salt

1. In a medium saucepan, melt the Coconut Bliss and coconut oil over medium heat. Add the chocolate and cook, stirring, until the chocolate has melted. Whisk in the vanilla, espresso, and salt and blend well. Remove from the heat and let cool to room temperature before using.

2. Pour any leftover sauce into a glass jar and refrigerate. The sauce will keep in the refrigerator for up to 3 months. Gently reheat until pourable before using.

Appendix A

Medicinal Uses for Cannabinoids

Cannabinoids definition (*noun*): a set of closely related chemicals unique to cannabis that constitute the active ingredients of the plant.

	THC	CBD	CBN	THC-A	
					Neurological
Concussion	X	X			
Epilepsy/Seizures	X	X	X	X	
Multiple Sclerosis	X	X	X	X	
Muscle Spasms	X	X			
Restless Leg Syndrome	X	X			
Stroke	X	X			
Tourette's Syndrome	X				
					Pain/Sleep
Arthritis	X	X	X	X	
Cramps	X	X			

Fibromyalgia	X	X		
Headaches/Migraine	X	X		
Insomnia	X	X	X	
Sleep Apnea	X			
Spinal Injury	X	X		
Gastrointestinal				
Anorexia	X	X		
Appetite Loss	X			
Crohn's Disease	X	X		X
Diabetes		X		
High Blood Pressure	X	X		
Nausea	X	X		
Mental Illness				
ADHD	X	X		
Anxiety		X		
Bipolar	X	X		
Depression	X	X	X	
OCD	X	X		
PTSD	X	X		
Other Illnesses				
Asthma	X			
Cancer	X	X		X
Chronic Immune System Disorders				X
Glaucoma	X			
HIV/AIDS	X			X
Opiate Addiction	X	X		

Appendix B

Online Resources

The following websites contain information about the health benefits of cannabis.

CANNABIS AND CANCER
http://www.thedailybeast.com/articles/2012/09/06/marijuana-fights-cancer-and-helps-manage-side-effects-researchers-find.html

CANNABIS AND NAUSEA
http://www.advancedholistichealth.org/PDF_Files/Regulation%20of%20nausea%20and%20vomiting%20by%20cannabinoids.pdf

CANNABIS AND PTSD
http://veteransformedicalmarijuana.org/content/general-use-cannabis-ptsd-symptoms

CANNABIS AND STROKE
http://www.huffingtonpost.co.uk/2013/12/03/cannabis-may-help-stroke-recovery_n_4376100.html

CENTER FOR MEDICINAL CANNABIS RESEARCH, UNIVERSITY OF SAN DIEGO, CALIFORNIA
http://www.cmcr.ucsd.edu/

DR. WILLIAM COURTNEY, CANNABIS INTERNATIONAL
http://www.cannabisinternational.org/about.php

DR. TIM ENGLAND
http://www.nottinghampost.com/Stroke-survivors-given-cannabis-reduce-brain/story
-20249666-detail/story.html

DR. SANJAY GUPTA, CNN MEDICAL CORRESPONDENT
http://www.cnn.com/2013/08/08/health/gupta-changed-mind-marijuana/index.html

DR. RAPHAEL MECHOULAM
http://israel21c.org/people/the-israeli-pharmacologist-who-kick-started-marijuana-research/

DR. ALAN SCHACKLEFORD
http://www.amarimed.com

ROBIN AND CHERI HACKETT, BOTANACARE
http://www.botanacare.com

SUMMARY OF RECENT RESEARCH ON MEDICAL MARIJUANA
http://norml.org/component/zoo/category/recent-research-on-medical-marijuana

Acknowledgments

With my love and thanks to:

My wonderful, supportive daughter, Lucienne O. Lazarus, and Gaetano Iannaccone, recipe testers extraordinaire who whipped, beat, scalded, torched, sliced, diced, flambéed, and baked every recipe, over and over until they reached perfection. Photographer Povy Atchison and food stylists Chad Forsberg and Lucienne O. Lazarus, for creating the stunning photographs. Gabrielle Campo, my editor, who guided me through, and who was there for me when I had no idea of what the next step should be. I feel lucky to have gotten to work with her. My agent, Marc Gerald, for believing in me from the get-go. He knew I could do it before I did. Karen Palmer, whose meticulous work and vast knowledge turned all my Post-its, scribbles, ramblings, and lists into a real book.

I am beyond indebted to the Sweet Mary Jane team: Grace Gutierrez, for her artistry, saintly patience, and organizational skills that continually floor me. Thomas Kee, for his eternal optimism and kitchen inspiration. Chad Forsberg, who bakes up batches of magic time and time again in the most graceful fashion and does it all with good cheer. Charley Bercow, for never saying no, no matter how hard the task. And there were many times I wondered how he did it. Alex Ivers, for his sweetness and dedication. Emily Sloat, for joining the Sweet Mary Jane team. Sweet Mary Jane's customers, without whom this bakery never would have become what it is today.

Robin and Cheri Hackett of Botanacare, for their kindness, love, and support. Robin, thank you for keeping me laughing throughout all the insanity. Danny Sloat and Evan Simons, who are the best cannabis growers I have ever met. Those buds you see in the photos? Yep, grown by these two guys. Ali Lansing, who makes our concentrates. Green Cross Couriers, who travel all over Colorado to deliver our confections.

My brother, Paul, for cheering me on. My dog, Maggie, who loyally sat by my desk every night, waiting patiently for me to finish typing and never once complained. My friends, who stood by me when I canceled every single brunch, dinner, concert, hike, and workout session.

And, finally, I would like to thank the people of Colorado, who in the spirit of freedom have given all of us who work in this industry the opportunity to realize our dreams.

Index

Page numbers in **bold** indicate tables; those in *italics* indicate photographs.

A

ADHD, 17, **280**
Adzuki Kooky Cupcakes, *150*, 151–53
Alex's Mint Madness, 60–61
Alice, 52–53, 58–59
almonds
   Black Sesame Cacao Nib Brittle, 222–23
   Blood Orange–Ginger Sweet Bread, *124*, 125–26
   Chocolate-Almond Delights, *218*, 219–21
   Gone Crackers, *230*, 231–32
   High-End Celestial Cookie, 39, *106*, 107–9
   Mark T's Raw Bar Yogi Treats, 85
   Queen of Tarts, *182*, 183–85
Aloha Truffles, *256*, 257–58

altitude baking, 22
Amendment 20 (Colorado), 5
anorexia, **280**
anxiety, 17, **280**
appetite loss, **280**
Apple Pie, Four-and-Twenty, 175–77
Apples, Baked Meringue Pomegranate, 235–36, *237*
apricots, High-End Celestial Cookie, 39, *106*, 107–9
arrowroot powder, 29
arthritis, 17, **279**
asthma, **280**
Aw, Snap! Margarita Brittle, 233–34, *234*

B

bacon, French Toast Cupcakes, 147–48
Baked Meringue Pomegranate Apples, 235–36, *237*
baking pans, 21–22
Baklava, Rosewater, 170–72
Banana–Double Chocolate Cupcakes with Fluffy Coconut Frosting, 144–46
bars and brownies, 8, 10, 57–85
Berry Entertaining Blueberry Coffee Cake, 127–28
Better Budder Peanut Butter Cookies, 88–89
Big Bhang! Cookies, *90*, 91–92
Big S Oatmeal Cookies, *114*, 115–16
bipolar, **280**
bittersweet chocolate, 30
   Caramel Sugar Highs, 224–26

bittersweet chocolate (*cont.*)
  Chocolate-Almond
    Delights, *218,* 219–21
  Chocolate Supremes, *96,*
    97–98
  Gone Crackers, *230,* 231–32
  High-End Celestial
    Cookie, 39, *106,* 107–9
  Lucie in the Sky, *102,*
    103–5, *104*
  Magic Moment Sauce, 276
  OMG! Brownie
    Cheesecake Bars, 4, 10,
    72, 73–75
  Queen of Tarts, *182,* 183–85
  Wicked Chocolate Sorbet,
    192
  Zo-Zo Snaps, 119–20
Black Sesame–Cacao Nib
  Brittle, 222–23
Blood Orange–Ginger Sweet
  Bread, *124,* 125–26
blueberries
  Berry Entertaining
    Blueberry Coffee Cake,
    127–28
  Blueberry-Peach Cobbler,
    173–74
  Pop Star Peanut Butter
    Parfait, *204,* 205
Bob's Red Mill All-Purpose
  Baking Flour, 31
Boulder, Colorado, 1, 3, 7,
  9, 85
Boulder Beer "Shake"
  Chocolate Porter, 160
Bourbon–Salted Caramel
  Sauce, 274

bowls, 22
Brittle, Aw, Snap! Margarita,
  233–34, *234*
Brittle, Black Sesame–Cacao
  Nib, 222–23
brownies and bars, 8, 10,
  57–85
brown sugar, 32
bud. *See* cannabis
Buddha Budda, 12, 24–25,
  29, 37, 41, 49, 51
Buddha Budda (recipe), *42,*
  43–45
butter, 29
  See also Buddha Budda
Buttercream Orange Filling
  and Frosting, 160, 161–62
butterscotch
  Big Bhang! Cookies, *90,*
    91–92
  Lick the Spoon!
    Butterscotch Pudding,
    208, 209–10
  Some Like It Hot
    Mexican-Spiced Fudge,
    238, 239–40

C

Cacao Nib–Black Sesame
  Brittle, 222–23
cacao nibs, 30
cake flour, 31
cakes and sweet breads,
  121–41
calculating doses, 40, 41,
  54–55
cancer, 17, 40, **280,** 281
candy thermometer, 22

cannabis, *20, 29, 36*
  calculating doses, 40, 41,
    54–55
  cannabinoids, 6, 17–18, *18,*
    38, **279–80**
  CBD, 17, 18, **279–80**
  CBN, 44, 45, 47, 48, 53,
    279–80
  children caution, 13, 40
  cooking, smelling like
    weed, 13
  doses, 12–13, 37–38, 40,
    41, 54–55
  *endo*cannabinoids, 6
  health benefits from, 4,
    6, 12, 15–18, 40, 46,
    279–80
  "high," 40
  legalization of, 5, 6, 11,
    12, 15
  oral (edible) vs. inhaled
    (smoked), 13, 17–18,
    37–39
  overdosing, 37–38
  quality of, 41
  Schedule I substance, 15–16
  strength (potency) of, 54
  sweet leaf, 49
  THC-A (Tetrahydrocan-
    nabinolic acid), 18, 40,
    41, **279–80**
  THC (Delta-9-
    tetrahydrocannabinol),
    7, 17, 18, 37, 38, 39,
    40–41, 54–55, **279–80**
  websites, 5, 281–82
  See also recipes
cannabis co-op, 11–12

Cannabis International, 15

"Cannabis Medicine in Perspective," 16

capric/caprylic acid, 46

caramel

    Caramel Buttercream Frosting, *164*, 165, 166–67

    Caramel Sugar Highs, 224–26

    Pop Star Caramel Corn, 8, 246–47

    Salted Caramel–Bourbon Sauce, 274

Carrot Cake Cookies, 4, 93–95, *95*

cashews, Pop Star Caramel Corn, 8, 246–47

cash problem, 11

CBD, 17, 18, **279–80**

CBN, 44, 45, 47, 48, 53, **279–80**

Celestial Cookie, High-End, 39, *106*, 107–9

Center for Medicinal Cannabis Research at University of California, San Diego, 15, 281

Chai High Truffles, 4, *256*, 259–60

Cheesecake Bars, OMG! Brownie, 4, 10, *72*, 73–75

cheesecloth, 24

children caution, 13, 40

Chocolate-Almond Delights, *218*, 219–21

Chocolate (Double)–Banana

Cupcakes with Fluffy Coconut Frosting, 144–46

Chocolate-Filled Pandan Dumplings, *5*

Chocolate Pastry Dough, *182*, 183, 184

chocolates, 8, 30

    See also specific chocolate

Chocolate Supremes, 96, 97–98

Chocolate Thunder, 131–32

Cinnamon Cream Cheese, 181

CNN, 15, 282

Cobbler, Blueberry-Peach, 173–74

cocoa powder, 30

Cocolove chocolate, 30

coconut

    Aloha Truffles, *256*, 257–58

    Coconut Cream Frosting, 153

    Cool It! Coconut-Vanilla Ice Cream, 193–94, *195*

    Double Chocolate-Banana Cupcakes with Fluffy Coconut Frosting, 144–46

    Fluffy Coconut Frosting, 144, 145, 146

    420 Matcha-Sama Truffles, *256*, 267–68

    French Kiss Toasted Macaroons, 117–18

Coconut Bliss, 12, 24–25, 31, 37, 41, 49, 51

Coconut Bliss (recipe), 46–48

coconut oil, 31

    See also Coconut Bliss

coffee, 31

coffee cakes

    Berry Entertaining Blueberry Coffee Cake, 127–28

    Just Peachy Coffee Cake, *134*, 135–36, *137*

    Mad Batter Chocolate Chip Coffee Cake, 129–30, *130*

coffee filters, 22

Colorado, 1, 3, 5, 6, 7, 9, 10, 11–12, 15, 16, 38, 39, 267

Compost Cookie, 91

concussions, 17, **279**

confections, art form, 3

    See also Lazarus, Karin; recipes

cookie cutter, 22–23

cookies, 8, 87–120

cooking and smelling like weed, 13

cooling racks, 26

Cool It! Coconut-Vanilla Ice Cream, 193–94, *195*

Courtney, William, 15, 281

Crackers, Gone, *230*, 231–32

cramps, **279**

cream cheese

    Carrot Cake Cookies, 4, 93–95, *95*

    Cheesy-Olive, Savory Pop Tarts, 181

    Cinnamon Cream Cheese, 181

cream cheese (*cont.*)

Cream Cheese Frosting, 111, 112

Matcha Green Tea Frosting, *150*, 151, 153

OMG! Brownie Cheesecake Bars, 4, 10, 72, *73*–75

Pop Rocks Sandwich Cookies, *110*, 111–13

creative bites, 217–53

Crème Brûlée, Vanilla Angel, 211–12, *213*

Crofters Organic Just Fruit Spread, 78

Crohn's disease, 17, **280**

crusts

cupcakes and muffins, *164*, 165, 166

Graham Cracker Crust, 73, 74

tarts and pastries, 175, 176, *186*, 187, 188

cupcakes and muffins, 143–67

D

dark chocolate

Aloha Truffles, 256, 257–58

Better Budder Peanut Butter Cookies, 88–89

Dark Chocolate Cupcakes, *150*, 151–53

420 Matcha-Sama Truffles, 256, 267–68

Late-Night Snack Truffles, 256, 263–64

Scout's Honor, 256, 269–70

decarboxylation, 25, 40–41

DeFloured menu, Sweet Mary Jane Bakery, 83

Delta-9-tetrahydrocannabinol (THC), 7, 17, 18, 37, 38, 39, 40–41, 54–55, **279–80**

depression, 17, **280**

diabetes, 17, **280**

Divine chocolate, 30

doses of THC, 12–13, 37–38, 40, 41, 54–55

dosing, keeping track of, 40, 41, 54–55

Double Chocolate–Banana Cupcakes with Fluffy Coconut Frosting, 144–46

dried fruits, 31

Alice, 52–53, 58–59

Carrot Cake Cookies, 4, 93–95, 95

Good Day Sunshine, *62*, 63–64

Lucie in the Sky, *102*, 103–5, *104*

Mark T's Raw Bar Yogi Treats, 85

Smashing Pumpkin Bars, *80*, 81–82

Drug Enforcement Administration, 15–16

Dutch-process cocoa powder (nonalkalized), 30

E

Ecstasy, 16

Ecstasy Sauce, *272*, 273

edible vs. inhaled cannabis, 13, 17–18, 37–39

eggs, 31

*endo*cannabinoids, 6

England, Tim, 17, 282

epilepsy/seizures, 17, **279**

equipment and terms, 12, 21–26

Espresso (Shot of) Muffins, 158–59

extracts, 31

F

Falkner, Elizabeth, 5

Farewell to Peaches, 227–28

Feel the Love Lemon Sandwich Cookies, 99–101

fibromyalgia, 17, **280**

flans and puddings, 207–16

flour, 31

Fluffy Coconut Frosting, 144, 145, 146

Food and Drug Administration, 15–16

food processor, 23

420 Matcha-Sama Truffles, 256, 267–68

Four-and-Twenty Apple Pie, 175–77

French Kiss Toasted Macaroons, 117–18

French Toast Cupcakes, 147–48

Frosted Flakes, Chocolate-Almond Delights, *218*, 219–21

frostings

Caramel Buttercream, *164*, 165, 166–67
Coconut Cream, 153
Cream Cheese, 111, 112
Fluffy Coconut, 144, 145, 146
Matcha Green Tea, *150*, 151, 153
Orange Buttercream, 160, 161–62
Sweet Cream, *154*, 155, 156, 157
fudge, Some Like It Hot Mexican-Spiced Fudge, *238*, 239–40

G

ganache, 31, 131, 132
gastrointestinal medicinal uses, 17, **280**
genetically modified organisms (GMOs), 29
Ginger–Blood Orange Sweet Bread, *124*, 125–26
Girl Scouts, 2, 269
glaucoma, 17, **280**
gluten-free baking, 31, 63, 83, 111, 117, 183
Gone Crackers, *230*, 231–32
Good Day Sunshine, *62*, 63–64
graham crackers
    Big Bhang! Cookies, *90*, 91–92
    Graham Cracker Crust, 73, 74
    Key Lime Kickers, 4, 10, *256*, 261–62

S'mores, 23, *248*, 249
granulated white sugar, 9, 32
    See also Hey Sugar!
Greek yogurt, Hops to It Cupcakes, 31, 160–62
grinder, 23
Grinspoon, Lester, 16
Gupta, Sanjay, 15, 282
Gutierrez, Grace, 239

H

Hackett, Robin and Cheri, 282
Harvard Mental Health Letter, 16
HB-1284 (Colorado), 5–6
headaches, **280**
head shops in New York City, 2
health benefits from cannabis, 4, 6, 12, 15–18, 40, 46, **279–80**
heavy cream
    Aloha Truffles, *256*, 257–58
    Caramel Sugar Highs, 224–26
    Chai High Truffles, 4, *256*, 259–60
    Chocolate-Almond Delights, *218*, 219–21
    Chocolate Thunder, 131–33
    Cool It! Coconut-Vanilla Ice Cream, 193–94, *195*
    Farewell to Peaches, 227–28
    420 Matcha-Sama Truffles, *256*, 267–68

ganache, 31, 131, 132
Key Lime Kickers, 4, 10, *256*, 261–62
Late-Night Snack Truffles, *256*, 263–64
Lavender Ice Cream, *196*, 197–98
Malted Milk Truffles, *256*, 265–66
Mind Eraser Parfaits, 202
Queen of Tarts, *182*, 183–85
Salted Caramel–Bourbon Sauce, 274
Scout's Honor, *256*, 269–70
Sweet Cream Frosting, *154*, 155, 156, 157
Vanilla Angel Crème Brûlée, 211–12, *213*
Whipped Cream, 227, 228
Hebrew University, Jerusalem, 15
helpful cooking measurement equivalents, 12, 26
Hemp Connoisseur THC Championship, 10, 261
heroin, 16
Hey Sugar!, 13, 23, 33, 37, 41
Hey Sugar! (recipe), *50*, 51–54, *52*
Hickenlooper, John (Colorado Governor), 12
"high," 40
high blood pressure, 17, **280**
High-End Celestial Cookie, 39, *106*, 107–9
high-percentage chocolate, 30
HIV/AIDS, 17, **280**
honey, 33

Hops to It Cupcakes, 31, 160–62
"hour of cannabis consumption," 267

I

ice cream maker, 23
ice creams and sorbets, 191–205
ilovesmj.com, 5
I Love You, Alice B. Toklas (movie), 5
immune system disorders, **280**
infusions, 9, 12, 35–55
    See also recipes
ingredients, 12, 29–33
inhaled vs. edible cannabis, 13, 17–18, 37–39
insomnia, **280**
insulin levels, 17
Ivers, Alex, 60

J

Just Peachy Coffee Cake, *134*, 135–36, *137*

K

Keebler Grasshoppers, Scout's Honor, 256, 269–70
Key Lime Kickers, 4, 10, *256*, 261–62
Kooky Adzuki Cupcakes, *150*, 151–53

L

lactose-intolerant, 83
Late-Night Snack Truffles, *256*, 263–64

lauric acid, 46
Lavender Ice Cream, *196*, 197–98
Lazarus, Karin, 1–13
    awards won by, 10, 261
    background of, 1–4
    ilovesmj.com, 5
    Lucienne (Karen's daughter), 3, 7, 103
    medical marijuana bakery, 4–12
    Sweet Mary Jane in Boulder, Colorado, 1, 4, 9–11, 18, 41, 60, 69, 73, 83, 111, 119, 239, 243, 246, 269
    See also cannabis; recipes
legalization of cannabis, 5, 6, 11, 12, 15
lemon
    Feel the Love Lemon Sandwich Cookies, 99–101
    Lemon Love Bars, 66, 67–68, *68*
    Tangy Lemon Curd Filling, 99
Lick the Spoon! Butterscotch Pudding, *208*, 209–10
LSD, 16
Lucie in the Sky, *102*, 103–5, *104*

M

macadamia nuts, Aloha Truffles, *256*, 257–58
Macaroons, French Kiss Toasted, 117–18
Mad Batter Chocolate Chip

Coffee Cake, 129–30, *130*
Magic Moment Sauce, 276
Malted Milk Truffles, *256*, 265–66
Mango Sweet Temptation Sorbet, *200*, 201
maple, Good Day Sunshine, 62, *63*–64
Maple-Pumpkin Moon Pies, *138*, 139–41
Margarita Brittle, Aw, Snap!, 233–34, *234*
marijuana. *See* cannabis
Marijuana Enforcement Division, 10
Marijuana for Medical Professional Conference in Denver, 16
Marijuana Infused Products license, 7
Marijuana Inventory Tracking System, 10–11
Marijuana Policy Project, 16
marking edibles clearly, 39
Mark T's Raw Bar Yogi Treats, 85
Marshmallows, Peppermint, *242*, 243–45
marshmallows, S'mores, 23, *248*, 249
marzipan, High-End Celestial Cookie, 39, *106*, 107–9
mason jars, 23
matcha green tea, 31
    420 Matcha-Sama Truffles, *256*, 267–68

Matcha Green Tea
    Frosting, *150*, 151, 153
measurement equivalents,
    12, 26
measuring cups, 23
Mechoulam, Raphael, 15,
    282
medical marijuana bakery,
    4–12
    See also Sweet Mary Jane
        in Boulder, Colorado
medium-chain triglycerides,
    46
mental illness medicinal uses,
    280
Merciful, 8, 69–70, *71*
Meringue Pomegranate
    Apples, Baked, 235–36,
    237
methamphetamine, 16
Mexican-Spiced Fudge, Some
    Like It Hot, *238*, 239–40
migraines, **280**
milk chocolate, 30
    Alex's Mint Madness,
        60–61
    Malted Milk Truffles, *256*,
        265–66
    Some Like It Hot
        Mexican-Spiced Fudge,
        238, 239–40
milligrams of THC,
    calculating, 40, 41, 54–55
Mind Eraser Parfaits, 202
Mint Madness, Alex's, 60–61
mise en place ("put in
    place"), 4, 21
mixer, 23

molasses, 33
Momofuko Milk Bar, 91
Moon Pies, Maple-Pumpkin,
    138, 139–41
muffins and cupcakes,
    143–67
multiple sclerosis, 17, **279**
muscle spasms, 17, 40, **279**

N

nausea, **280**, 281
neurological medicinal uses,
    16–17, **279**
New York City, 2–3, 6
NORML, 16, 282
Nutella, S'mores, 23, *248*,
    249
nuts. *See specific nuts*

O

Oatmeal Cookies, Big S, *114*,
    115–16
OCD, **280**
offset spatula, 24
OMG! Brownie Cheesecake
    Bars, 4, 10, *72*, 73–75
opiate addiction, 17, **280**
oral (edible) vs. inhaled
    (smoked) cannabis, 13,
    17–18, 37–39
Orange Buttercream Filling
    and Frosting, 160,
    161–62
overdosing, 37–38

P

pain/sleep medicinal uses, 17,
    279–80

paint strainers, 24
palliative effects of
    cannabis, 17
parchment paper, 24
Parfait, Pop Star Peanut
    Butter, *204*, 205
Parfaits, Mind Eraser, 202
pastries and tarts, 169–89
pastry bags and tips, 24
patient, being, 38–39
peaches
    Blueberry-Peach Cobbler,
        173–74
    Farewell to Peaches,
        227–28
    Just Peachy Coffee Cake,
        134, 135–36, *137*
peanut butter
    Better Budder Peanut
        Butter Cookies,
        88–89
    Pop Star Peanut Butter
        Parfait, *204*, 205
    Silky Sweet Peanut Butter
        Sauce, 275
    True Confections, 8, *250*,
        251–53, *252*
Pear Tart, Sweetie Pie, *186*,
    187–89, *188*
pecans
    Chocolate Supremes, *96*,
        97–98
    Farewell to Peaches,
        227–28
    Just Peachy Coffee Cake,
        134, 135–36, *137*
    Smashing Pumpkin Bars,
        80, 81–82

peppermint, Alex's Mint Madness, 60–61
Peppermint Marshmallows, *242*, 243–45
peyote, 16
phyllo dough, Rosewater Baklava, 170–72
pie weights, 24
pistachio nuts
  Chocolate Thunder, 131–33
  High-End Celestial Cookie, 39, *106*, 107–9
  Rose Petal Sweet Bread, 122–23
  Rosewater Baklava, 170–72
Pomegranate Apples, Baked Meringue, 235–36, *237*
popcorn, Pop Star Caramel Corn, 8, 246–47
Pop Rocks Sandwich Cookies, *110*, 111–13
Pop Star Caramel Corn, 8, 246–47
Pop Star Peanut Butter Parfait, *204*, 205
Pop Tarts, *178*, 179–81
porter beer, Hops to It Cupcakes, 31, 160–62
potato chips, Big Bhang! Cookies, *90*, 91–92
potato chips, Late-Night Snack Truffles, *256*, 263–64
potency (strength) of cannabis, 54
powdered sugar (confectioners' sugar, icing sugar), 33

pretzels
  Big Bhang! Cookies, *90*, 91–92
  Late-Night Snack Truffles, *256*, 263–64
  True Confections, *250*, 251–53, *252*
PTSD, 17, **280**, 281
puddings and flans, 207–16
pumpkin
  Aw, Snap! Margarita Brittle, 233–34, *234*
  Maple-Pumpkin Moon Pies, *138*, 139–41
  Pumpkin Flan with Pumpkin Seed Praline, 214–16
  Smashing Pumpkin Bars, *80*, 81–82
Pyrex dishes, 24

Q

quality of cannabis, 41
Queen of Tarts, *182*, 183–85

R

Raisin Rum Cupcakes, *154*, 155–57
Raspberry Jam Session, *76*, 77–78
Raw Bar Yogi Treats, Mark T's, 85
raw food movement, 85
raw sugar, 33
recipes
  altitude baking, 22
  brownies and bars, 8, 10, 57–85

cakes and sweet breads, 121–41
cookies, 8, 87–120
creative bites, 217–53
cupcakes and muffins, 143–67
equipment and terms, 12, 21–26
helpful cooking measurement equivalents, 12, 26
ice creams and sorbets, 191–205
infusions, 9, 12, 35–55
ingredients, 12, 29–33
puddings and flans, 207–16
sauces, 271–76
servings and milligrams of THC in, 40, 41, 54–55
sweeteners, 32–33
tarts and pastries, 169–89
testing recipes, 8–9, 73
truffles, 8, 256–70
  See also cannabis; Lazarus, Karin
Red Cards, 6
regulations, keeping up with, 10–11
restless leg syndrome, 17, **279**
rolled oats
  Big Bhang! Cookies, *90*, 91–92
  Big S Oatmeal Cookies, *114*, 115–16
  Good Day Sunshine, *62*, 63–64
  Lucie in the Sky, *102*, 103–5, *104*

Mark T's Raw Bar Yogi
    Treats, 85
Raspberry Jam Session, 76,
    77–78
Rooster THC Classic, 10
Rose Petal Sweet Bread,
    122–23
rosewater, 32
Rosewater Baklava, 170–72
Royal Derby Hospital, 17
rubber gloves, 24–25
ruler, 25
Rum Raisin Cupcakes, 154,
    155–57

S

Salted Caramel–Bourbon
    Sauce, 274
San Rafael, California, 267
sauces, 271–76
Savory Pop Tarts, 178, 179–81
scale, 25
Schackleford, Alan, 282
Scharffen Berger Chocolate,
    5, 30
Schedule I substance, 15–16
Scout's Honor, 256, 269–70
seeds, Good Day Sunshine,
    62, 63–64
seeds, Mark T's Raw Bar
    Yogi Treats, 85
semisweet chocolate, 30
    Big Bhang! Cookies, 90,
        91–92
    Chocolate Supremes, 96,
        97–98
    Chocolate Thunder, 131–33
    ganache, 31, 131, 132

Lucie in the Sky, 102,
    103–5, 104
Mad Batter Chocolate
    Chip Coffee Cake,
    129–30, 130
Magic Moment Sauce, 276
Merciful, 8, 69–70, 71
    Shot of Espresso Muffins,
        158–59
Sensible Colorado, 16
servings and milligrams of
    THC in, 40, 41, 54–55
Sesame (Black)–Cacao Nib
    Brittle, 222–23
Shot of Espresso Muffins,
    158–59
silicone baking mats, 24
Silky Sweet Peanut Butter
    Sauce, 275
sleep apnea, 280
Smashing Pumpkin Bars, 80,
    81–82
smelling like weed and
    cooking, 13
smoked vs. edible cannabis,
    13, 17–18, 37–39
S'mores, 23, 248, 249
sober, baking, 39
Some Like It Hot Mexican-
    Spiced Fudge, 238,
    239–40
sorbets and ice creams,
    191–205
sour cream, Four-and-
    Twenty Apple Pie,
    175–77
spices, 32
spinal injury, 280

"Start low. Go slow," 39
stoned, don't bake when, 39
"stoner food," 8
stout beer, Hops to It
    Cupcakes, 31, 160–62
strainers, 25
strength (potency) of
    cannabis, 54
stroke, 17, 279, 281
sugar, infused granulated
    white, 9, 32
    See also Hey Sugar!
sweet breads and cakes,
    121–41
Sweet Cream Frosting, 154,
    155, 156
sweeteners, 32–33
Sweetie Pie Pear Tart, 186,
    187–89, 188
sweet leaf, 49
Sweet Mary Jane in Boulder,
    Colorado, 1, 4, 9–11, 18,
    41, 60, 69, 73, 83, 111,
    119, 239, 243, 246, 269
    See also Lazarus, Karin
Sweet Pop Tarts, 178, 179–81
Sweet Temptation Mango
    Sorbet, 200, 201

T

Tangy Lemon Curd Filling, 99
tarts and pastries, 169–89
tasting as you cook caution, 13
temperature gun (laser
    thermometer), 25
tequila, Aw, Snap! Margarita
    Brittle, 233–34, 234
testing recipes, 8–9, 73

THC-A (Tetrahydro
cannabinolic acid), 18,
40, 41, **279–80**
THC (Delta-9-
tetrahydrocannabinol),
7, 17, 18, 37, 38, 39,
40–41, 54–55, **279–80**
Thin Mints, Scout's Honor,
256, 269–70
thin wooden skewers, 25
timer, 25
tolerance of THC, 38, 39
*Tonight Show Starring
Jimmy Fallon, The* (TV
show), 155
toothpicks, 25
torch, 25
tortilla chips, Aw, Snap!
Margarita Brittle,
233–34, *234*
Tortola, British Virgin
Islands, 3, 5
Tosi, Christina, 91
Tourette's syndrome, 17, **279**
True Confections, 8, *250*,
251–53, *252*
truffles, 8, 256–70
TuttiFoodie, 5
Twix Tricks Cupcakes, *164*,
165–67

U

University of California, San
Diego, 15, 281
University of Nottingham,
17, 282
unsweetened chocolate, 30

Chocolate Pastry Dough,
182, 183, 184
Dark Chocolate Cupcakes,
150, 151–53
Ecstasy Sauce, *272*, 273
Hops to It Cupcakes, 31,
160–62
Kooky Adzuki Cupcakes,
150, 151–53
Mark T's Raw Bar Yogi
Treats, 85
Merciful, 8, 69–70, *71*
Twix Tricks Cupcakes,
164, 165–67
Walnut Fantasy, 8, 83–84

V

vanilla, 32
Cool It! Coconut-Vanilla
Ice Cream, 193–94, *195*
Vanilla Angel Crème
Brûlée, 211–12, *213*
vanilla ice cream, *196*,
197–98
vegan baking, 63, 85
vegetable shortening, 32

W

"Waldos, The," 267
walnuts
Baked Meringue
Pomegranate Apples,
235–36, *237*
Chocolate Supremes, *96*,
97–98
Four-and-Twenty Apple
Pie, 175–77

OMG! Brownie
Cheesecake Bars, 4, 10,
72, 73–75
Rosewater Baklava,
170–72
Some Like It Hot
Mexican-Spiced Fudge,
238, 239–40
Walnut Fantasy, 8,
83–84
websites, 5, 281–82
weed. *See* cannabis
Weeds (TV show), 4
white chocolate, 30
Alice, 52–53, 58–59
Chai High Truffles, 4,
256, 259–60
Chocolate-Almond
Delights, *218*,
219–21
Key Lime Kickers, 4, 10,
256, 261–62
Smashing Pumpkin Bars,
80, 81–82
True Confections, 8, *250*,
251–53, *252*
Wicked Chocolate Sorbet,
192
wire cooling racks, 26
wooden skewers, 25

Y

Yogi Treats, Mark T's Raw
Bar, 85

Z

Zo-Zo Snaps, 119–20